# sexually transmitted infections

the facts

# also available in the series

# sexually transmitted infections

## the facts

DAVID BARLOW M.A., B.M., B.Ch., F.R.C.P.,
F.R.C.P., (Edin), Hon F.C.V. Sri Lanka
Consultant Physician, Department of Genitourinary Medicine,
Guy's and St Thomas' Foundation Trust
Honorary Senior Lecturer,
United Medical and Dental Schools

'HIV and AIDS: the clinical picture' with
ALI MEARS M.B., M.R.C.O.G.,
Dip GUM, D.F.F.P.
Specialist Registrar, Department of Genitourinary Medicine,
Guy's and St Thomas' Foundation Trust

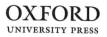

OXFORD
UNIVERSITY PRESS

# OXFORD

UNIVERSITY PRESS

Great Clarendon Street, Oxford OX2 6DP

Oxford University Press is a department of the University of Oxford.
It furthers the University's objective of excellence in research, scholarship,
and education by publishing worldwide in

Oxford New York

Auckland Cape Town Dar es Salaam Hong Kong Karachi
Kuala Lumpur Madrid Melbourne Mexico City Nairobi
New Delhi Shanghai Taipei Toronto

With offices in

Argentina Austria Brazil Chile Czech Republic France Greece
Guatemala Hungary Italy Japan Poland Portugal Singapore
South Korea Switzerland Thailand Turkey Ukraine Vietnam

Oxford is a registered trade mark of Oxford University Press
in the UK and in certain other countries

Published in the United States
by Oxford University Press Inc., New York

British Library Cataloguing in Publication Data

Data available

Library of Congress Cataloging in Publication Data

Barlow, David, F.R.C.P.
    Sexually transmitted infections : the facts / David Barlow.—2nd ed.
        p. cm.
    Includes bibliographical references and index.
    1. Sexually transmitted diseases.   I. Title.
RC200.2.B37 2006
616.95'1—dc22

                            2005028207

Typeset by Newgen Imaging Systems (P) Ltd., Chennai, India
Printed in Great Britain
on acid-free paper by
Clays Ltd., Bungay, Suffolk

ISBN 0–19–856867–3 (Pbk.)    978–0–19–856867–4

1

# preface

The first edition of this volume was published 27 years ago and a multitude of changes has occurred since then. In 1979, while headlines talked of the 'love virus', as herpes was labelled, no one was aware that another more deadly virus was spreading rapidly and inexorably from central Africa via Haiti to the East and then West coasts of North America. Although infection with the human immunodeficiency virus (HIV) was not to be recognized for another two years (and not named as such for a further four), this 'silent' period, akin to the latent period of the virus itself, allowed an insidious, lethal infection to infiltrate and establish itself in its first Western target group, gay men.

Aside from HIV infection, incidence of the other sexually transmitted diseases has changed (invariably upward) and the emphasis has shifted from bacterial infections to viral ones, warranting separate chapters for genital herpes and genital warts in this new edition. We should wonder at the new drugs that have become available, easier to take, more effective and often with fewer side-effects. There are new antivirals, new antifungals and new antibacterial preparations, many, however, remaining beyond the budget of developing economies. We should also wonder at the new diagnostic tools that are used – a quick 'pee-and-go' urine test replacing the infamous 'bottle-brush' for chlamydial and gonococcal infections in men. However, convenience may come at the price of false positives and negatives. A short chapter takes you through the pitfalls of interpreting these and other results.

Vaginal discharge, such a common symptom and still so often a source of misery, has yielded up some important secrets. In 1979 I wrote of 'non-specific vaginitis' caused by *Haemophilus vaginalis*. A year later this bacterium was renamed *Gardnerella vaginalis* while the condition briefly became 'anaerobic vaginosis' and then 'bacterial vaginosis' (BV) in the early 1980s. That decade witnessed the identification of the multitude of other bacteria responsible for the symptoms of BV and a better understanding of the factors that make this most common of conditions likely to occur and recur.

Our knowledge of human papilloma virus infection (HPV), responsible for warts both plain and genital, has expanded along with the introduction of topical treatments that promise to lighten the clinical and personal load of managing this common infection. How common? New diagnostic tools, using techniques of molecular biology, demonstrate that a majority of sexually active 25-year-old women are already infected with HPV. Thankfully, most of them do not go on to develop clinical warts. As we go to press, successful vaccines have been developed against two of the most important types of HPV.

Human immunodeficiency virus is included because it is primarily a sexually transmitted condition but this book cannot provide a comprehensive review of HIV infection and AIDS; for that there are other reference sources. We can all learn from an understanding of how and why the disease spread in the way it did, and from the (slow) development of tolerance for those particularly affected. I am grateful to have had the assistance of Dr Ali Mears in writing the section on the medical aspects of HIV infection; she is an able and knowledgeable clinician.

In 1979, my clinic at St Thomas' Hospital coped with 12 000 attendances. In 2006, some 45 000 pairs of feet will cross our threshold but will endure waiting times as unacceptable today as they would have been unthinkable 27 years ago. Annual attendance at GUM clinics in the UK has trebled and we are currently witnessing a resurgence of the 'classical' venereal diseases, gonorrhoea and syphilis, as well as record numbers of new cases of chlamydial infection. In spite of which gloom, there is still available in Great Britain the best service for the diagnosis and treatment of sexually transmitted diseases to be found anywhere in the world.

I hope this new edition will put the disease prevalence in perspective and help those who have, or think they have, or want to know how to avoid, or even just wish to know more about, sexually transmitted diseases, to adopt a calm approach to what is, these days, an eminently manageable group of conditions.

# acknowledgements

I would like to express my thanks to Melanie MacFarlane, Senior Nursing Sister in the Department of Genitourinary Medicine at Guy's and St Thomas' Hospitals, who in spite of pressures from babies and husband, to say nothing of a large department to run, made time to read through this manuscript and make important observations for improving its quality and accuracy. Her useful comments have been incorporated into the final draft. Many other members of staff have read odd little sections and I thank them for hiding their look of resignation as I approached them yet again for an opinion. Sylvia Wilkinson was good enough to read the manuscript and her suggestions have, I hope, made the final versions more accessible to the general reader. I finally thank my wife, Angela, for supporting me as I typed and my four grandchildren, Helena, Ella, Francesca, and Max for being somewhat short-changed during a six-month period.

# reviews of the first edition

Dr Barlow has written an excellent book. It is factual, short and witty. The book is aimed at a wide audience and is an important addition to the range of books on the subject. It is enjoyable and contains a description of all the important issues in modern genitourinary medicine. *The Lancet*

Barlow has a great deal to teach all doctors; it ought to be in every school and public library. The author pays us the complement of writing in plain English. Buy, borrow or steal it, you won't find my copy on the second-hand market. *World Medicine*

This book on sexually transmitted diseases will be of interest to a wide range of readers including health educators. Chapters on each of the infections contain a wealth of information. This book will be a welcome addition to libraries in schools, colleges for further education and teaching hospitals and will help to overcome the stigma of attending a hospital for treatment of diseases of a sexual nature. *British Journal of Venereal Diseases*

# contents

# introduction

This book is written from a United Kingdom perspective and although the diseases remain the same throughout the world, their incidence and relative importance varies considerably, as do the methods for delivery of care.

We are lucky in the UK to have a separate specialty of Genitourinary Medicine dating back to the early 1920s (then known as Venereology) with a reasonably well-funded network of clinics. The recognition of this specialty has brought with it a defined career structure which encourages young doctors who have already gained some years of general medical, surgical and gynaecological experience, to undergo further training which takes at least four years.

Apart from the Republic of Ireland, the only country with such an emphasis on the specialty is Australia, with training and central management of sexual health clinics organized by the Australasian College of Sexual Health Physicians. There are clinics in all areas, with large cities, like Sydney, having more than one. Examination and treatment are free. Most GPs have training in STIs and HIV infection is largely managed in primary care by GPs with special experience. This can be advantageous in terms of confidentiality since an Australian can attend any GP without needing to be registered with that particular practitioner.

Finding where to go for help is easy in Great Britain, Eire or Australia. In North America the City clinics are to be found in a telephone directory under 'VD' or 'sexually transmitted diseases/infections'. In Europe the specialty of dermato-venereology deals with sexually transmitted infections (STIs) but the large majority of specialists have skin diseases as their main interest. In Northern Europe there may be 'polyclinics' which concentrate on STIs and in all countries there will be some dermato-venereologists who have a special interest.

I suggest resource websites at the end of the chapters most of which include the British Association for Sexual Health and HIV (BASHH). In several areas the reader may find my advice or interpretation differs from the standard. If in doubt, it is best to consult your local GUM clinic. The quoted resources are mainly in the UK but are, obviously, accessible from overseas.

# 1 Sexually transmitted infections: what to do

There is a network of over 300 genitourinary medicine (GUM) clinics in the UK, which provide a service for matters related to sexual health and are staffed by health professionals, including doctors, nurses and health advisers. Only the Republic of Ireland, of all other countries, recognizes GUM as a distinct medical specialty. In other parts of the world, sexually transmitted infections (STIs) are managed by different specialties, including gynaecology (concerned with women's health), urology (concerned with kidney and bladder), andrology (concerned with men's health), infectious diseases and, most commonly, dermato-venereology, a specialty that combines skin diseases with sexually transmitted conditions. Dermato-venereologists are the predominant providers of service in Europe.

GUM clinics see the vast majority of STIs in the UK but perform a wider service than that. One of their important roles is in *excluding* STIs and reassuring people that they are not infected. For instance, the majority of HIV test results (and most of these are negative) are given in GUM clinics.

## What might I have caught?

'Germs' come in different sizes, the smallest of which are the viruses. These micro-organisms are so small that they are incapable of independent existence and replication unless they are inside a living cell. Some viruses can survive for periods away from cells but cannot grow or reproduce until they have infected a new host. Herpes simplex and the germs causing warts are viruses. Bacteria are larger than viruses and most can survive away from their host and even multiply. *Treponema pallidum* and *Neisseria gonorrhoeae* are bacteria. Next up in size comes *Trichomonas vaginalis*, which is a single-celled organism, called a protozoon. Larger still are the parasites, *Phthirus pubis*, causing crab louse infestation, and *Sarcoptes scabeii*, which causes scabies.

# Where to go?

For those uncertain about their genital symptoms, the first stop, after a chat with your mates in the pub, is likely to be the family doctor. The general practitioner (GP) is ideally placed to advise those worried about the possibility of a sexually transmitted infection. Most family practices will have a nurse with special training in sexual health who can advise on questions of family planning, cervical smear tests and STIs. The nurse will also be competent to take samples for laboratory investigations and will have special experience in the worries and potential problems concerning confidentiality.

The upside of the GP consultation is that you are dealing with a familiar face who knows your health background, in familiar surroundings, conveniently situated. The downside is that you are dealing with a familiar face who probably knows the rest of your family and may even be a family friend. You may not wish to share your problem under these circumstances.

# Why go to a GUM clinic?

The obvious anonymity of a hospital department may not seem so inviting when one is attending the only GUM clinic in a small town, its entrance, clearly sign-posted, leading off the main street. Most clinics, however, are strategically better placed and tend to be named after long forgotten heroes such as 'Martha and Luke' or 'James Pringle', or eminent venereologists of old, the Harrison Wing, the Claude Nicol Centre, rather than a bald 'Clap clinic this way'. The emphasis is on discretion. In the bad old days, the 'special' clinic was hidden, often in a basement, and decidedly away from the main, 'nice' parts of the hospital. Whatever its name, wherever its situation, the GUM clinic is designed and run to respect and maintain confidentiality, and these days they are mostly found within the main body of the hospital.

All doctors are bound by a duty of confidentiality but this has extra force in GUM clinics enshrined by an Act of Parliament incorporating the 'NHS Trusts and Primary Care Trusts (Sexually Transmitted Diseases) Directions 2000'. I quote:

> Every . . . Trust shall take all necessary steps to secure that any information capable of identifying an individual obtained by any of their members or employees with respect to persons examined or treated for any sexually transmitted disease shall not be disclosed except [and I paraphrase] to another health care professional also involved in their care or to prevent spread.

So, your details and the details of any infections are safeguarded by law. Even attendance at a clinic is kept secret, so the innocent telephone call, 'Can I have a word with my wife, Mrs Smith; I know she's there?', will be answered with a negative that neither acknowledges Mrs Smith's presence nor whether she is even a patient at the clinic.

Thus, reassuringly, everything that takes place within the clinic is confidential and patient records are kept separately from the ordinary hospital notes. This is one of the reasons why more people with HIV infection in the UK are looked after by genitourinary physicians, for both outpatient and inpatient care, than by other specialists.

Consultation and treatment are free and there is no need for a referral from a GP or other doctor.

You will be asked for personal details including name, date of birth and address. It is quite acceptable to insist on no contact at home and some attenders simply fail to give any address and give a false name. That is fine as long as the patient remembers the name they have given. On the books in our department, we have over seventy 'John Smiths', some of them no doubt genuine, fifteen 'Mickey Mouses' and a round dozen 'Donald Ducks'.

The other advantages of attending a clinic relate to its personnel, economy of scale and diagnostic facilities. Even in the smallest clinic there will be a specialist nurse and health adviser as well as the doctor, and in the majority there will be a larger team whose combined expertise cannot be achieved in other settings. There will be a larger range of potential investigations than is feasible at a GP's surgery with the great advantage that it is often possible to get the correct diagnosis and treatment at the time of first attendance. This is because various samples (such as vaginal discharge or urethral discharge) can be taken and examined on the spot, sometimes after staining with coloured dyes and using a microscope. Gonorrhoea, syphilis, non-specific urethritis (NSU), thrush, bacterial vaginosis and *Trichomonas vaginalis* are all diagnosable in this way, although the success rate of instant diagnosis does vary depending on the disease.

Finding other people who may also be infected (contact tracing) is a crucial part of the work of a GUM clinic, and partner notification is handled sensitively as a co-operation between patients and clinic staff.

## What investigations will I have?

This will depend very much on your reasons for attending. There is a list of standard tests that are done for those who attend just for a check-up. These should include blood tests for syphilis and HIV; I say 'tests', but only one blood sample is actually taken which is then split in the laboratory for the different analyses. Men and women will both be tested for chlamydial infection and gonorrhoea, and women will usually have samples looked at for three vaginal conditions: thrush, bacterial vaginosis and *Trichomonas vaginalis*, the only one of the three that is sexually transmitted.

The above would be a standard set of tests for an asymptomatic person attending before embarking on a new sexual relationship. Other tests including special ones for syphilis or herpes are not routine and will be done only if indicated by clinical findings or a patient's story. Usually a woman's urine will be tested and a mid-stream urine sample (MSU) sent off to the laboratory when there are urinary symptoms, pain or frequency passing urine, suggestive of a urinary tract infection (UTI).

In GUM clinics that cover the whole range of the specialty, smear tests and colposcopy (see Chapter 8) are available with dedicated clinics dealing with psychosexual problems, contraception, genital skin conditions and other specialist problems.

Homosexual men attending a clinic have their own different range of tests which simply reflects the fact that some infections are found more commonly than in heterosexuals. For example, tests for hepatitis A and B (Chapter 10) should be a routine unless there is a good history of vaccination.

## What if I am too young?

There are no restrictions on age, at either end of the scale, for those wishing to attend although the very young will, for obvious reasons, be accompanied by a parent or guardian. Those under the age of consent, 16 in the UK, do not need to have an older relative present and their confidentiality will be respected just as that of anyone else who attends.

## What happens when I attend a GUM clinic?

Attendance at a GUM clinic is often by appointment only but most clinics will see people who have an emergency ('my (now ex-) partner says he has given me gonorrhoea') on the same day. Some clinics maintain an open-access, no-appointment system, which can mean longer waiting times but does guarantee same-day consultation once (and if) registration has taken place. In some clinics there are different locations or times for the different sexes, in others there is a common waiting area and no distinction is made apart from the examination facilities for women. After booking-in, for both sexes there may be a triage in which the special needs of each patient are assessed, usually by a nurse, before they are channelled towards, say, a quick screening service or a slower medical assessment.

The medical history is taken usually by a doctor or, increasingly these days, by a nurse practitioner or nurse consultant. Whoever asks the questions, you will be reassured to know that they have heard it all before. For many people this will be the first time they have talked seriously about sex with anyone. Shame, embarrassment, anger, guilt, all of these may influence a person's attitude to what seem like particularly personal lines of questioning. Try to remember that, when you are asked whether you had oral sex with your boyfriend/girlfriend five nights ago, it is not idle curiosity that prompts the question, rather a need to know whether there is a possibility of, say, genital herpes (Chapter 7).

## What happens to a woman in a GUM clinic?

Once the history has been taken, which will include details of your menstrual cycle and obstetric history, you will be offered an examination which starts with a look at the vulva and pubic region and will then usually include passing a speculum into the vagina. It is the prospect of this examination that seems to fill many women with terror, even to the point where it provides the reason for putting off attendance. If the examination is done gently and slowly there is no need for discomfort or pain, but it certainly helps if the woman herself is relaxed.

The Cusco's speculum, which dates back to the eighteenth century, is the most commonly used instrument. It has two, rather unfortunately named, 'blades', hinged at one end and is oval or vulva-shaped at the other, ostensibly to facilitate passage into the vagina. It is common practice to twist the speculum once inserted, through 90° before opening the two halves. The entrance to the vagina is designed to receive a cylindrical object, the penis, and it has always surprised me how this uncomfortable twisting movement has stayed part of usual practice. Cusco designed his speculum to be used with the handles between the buttocks and this is certainly more comfortable than the common position with the handle by the clitoris where a slight nudge can be predictably uncomfortable. Before inserting the speculum the experienced operator will make sure that the wider, external, end of the speculum is warm, as well as the blades, as this is the bit in contact with the most sensitive parts. Disposable plastic speculums are often used these days but are inferior to the metal ones as they tend to 'stick' to the skin.

Using a cotton-tipped swab, samples are taken from the vagina and the cervix and are then either examined using the microscope, having been stained to show up different cells or micro-organisms, or sent off to the laboratory for culture or other forms of identification. 'Taking a sample' sounds as if it might be painful or uncomfortable. It isn't. Try rubbing a cotton bud gently across the back of your hand and that will reproduce exactly the pressure and feeling.

If gonorrhoea is being excluded samples will need to be taken from the urethra and rectum in women. In 5 per cent of cases, gonorrhoea will only be found in the urethra and in 5 per cent only in the rectum (Chapter 4) so, if these two sites are not checked, 10 per cent of cases will be missed. The rectal positive cases do not necessarily follow from rectal intercourse (although they might), as gonorrhoea can find its way into the back passage carried by a combination of gravity and the general moistness of the area. Both urethral and rectal samples are taken by passing a 'blind' swab into either orifice. This can be slightly uncomfortable in the urethra, but the rectal sample is usually described just as 'feeling a bit strange'.

After the speculum examination and urethral and rectal tests (if taken), a bimanual examination may follow. This is particularly important if there is a history of pain in the pelvic area, lower abdomen, or deep pain during intercourse. In a bimanual, one or two fingers of one hand are inserted into the vagina while the other, usually left, hand feels the lower abdomen (hence *bimanual*, two hands). In this way, using both hands the doctor can determine the outline, shape and size of any contents of the pelvis. They can assess whether there is evidence of pelvic inflammatory disease, fibroids in the uterus or see whether the uterus is enlarged when pregnancy is suspected. Once the examination is finished, any local measures can be applied including treatment for warts or molluscum contagiosum (Chapter 10).

After she has dressed, the female patient will be asked to wait while the various samples that have been taken are examined with the microscope. Causes of vaginal discharge or itching or smell are those most easily diagnosed on the spot using a combination of clinical examination and the microscope. Gonorrhoea, if present, will be found in less than half of cases (the others being diagnosed after culture of the bug in the laboratory).

If the tests are negative at the time of the initial examination, it is a good idea to ask the doctor whether they think there is likely to be any infection or what they believe may be the cause of your symptoms. The important thing to remember is that a definitive diagnosis cannot be made until the laboratory investigations have been completed and the fact that nothing has been found at the time of the first visit does not mean there is no infection.

# What happens to a man in a GUM clinic?

A man's progression through the clinic differs only in detail from that of the woman. Like her, he will be asked about his recent sexual encounters, whether a condom was used and if so, whether throughout intercourse. Questions regarding a partner's origin might appear offensive but such information can be vital when deciding on treatment. For example, gonorrhoea originating in the Philippines is much less easy to manage than gonorrhoea from Philadelphia.

After the history, the doctor examine the penis and, if relevant, the anus, for sores, spots, swellings or evidence of discharge. The foreskin will be retracted in the uncircumcised man to see if there are any untoward signs on the glans or the inside of the foreskin. Warts not uncommonly lurk at this site. The contents of the scrotum will be scrutinized; testes, epididymis and cords, which may be a rare chance for a man to have this sort of examination. Ideally a man should regularly examine his testicles for unusual lumps just as a woman should her breasts.

Today there are tests for chlamydia and gonorrhoea that can be performed simply on a sample of urine. These are fine as screening tests because they are sensitive and will usually pick up infection if it is there. There are, however, genuine problems with false positives (Chapter 2) and they do not pick up non-chlamydial urethritis, NSU, which is probably the most common diagnosis made in men attending the GUM clinic. For this, and to diagnose gonorrhoea on the spot, a urethral sample needs to be taken.

Because urinating tends to wash out the urethra, and because the urethra can be such a rich source of diagnostic material, the sample will be more useful if the patient has held his urine for at least three hours.

A thin plastic or platinum loop is gently inserted up to two centimetres into the urethra and any resulting discharge can be put on a microscope slide and examined. At the same time part of the discharge is sent to the laboratory on a special culture plate. If rectal intercourse has taken place samples will also be taken from the rectum for microscopy and culture.

If syphilis is suspected, a 'dark-ground' or 'dark-field' examination can be performed on fluid (serum) from a sore or rash. The sore is gently scraped and any fluid that exudes is examined microscopically. The sores are relatively painless and this procedure, like the urethral investigation, need give no cause for alarm. In general, men are luckier than women in that they are more likely to leave the clinic with a diagnosis at the end of their first visit.

# What if I have HIV infection?

Most people who come to the clinic do not have HIV infection and, accordingly, most of the HIV tests performed are negative. In the UK (see Chapter 11) those most at risk of HIV infection are homosexual men and heterosexual men or women from sub-Saharan Africa. We see a small number of injecting drug users (IDUs) but the predicted explosion of infection in this group has failed to materialize. At the time of writing (mid-2005), there is not a significant amount of transmission of HIV occurring in this country between heterosexuals.

Whatever the sexual orientation, geographical origin, or colour, there is one certainty in the UK: it is better to test than not to test. Chapter 12 explains the reasons in some detail but, in essence, today's management is so much better than yesterday's that HIV infection can be controlled in almost all cases – but only once the diagnosis has been made. All GUM clinics have facilities for HIV testing and experienced staff to explain all the processes. The message is simple: If in doubt, test!

# How can I use this book to find out if I have an infection?

The quick answer is that you should pop down to your local clinic and clear the matter up, once and for all. But, in real life you don't want to waste your time so we shall try to point you towards a likely, or at least possible, diagnosis, without having to leave your armchair.

The list of infections passed on by or during sexual activity seems to grow year by year. It is true that an even larger number of diseases can be passed on by close proximity with an infected person, for example, the common cold or tuberculosis, which no one would claim as predominantly sexually transmitted. However, common sense (and medical experience) suggests that, if, after having had sex with someone with a cold, you start to sneeze and sniffle, it is more likely to be a cold than chlamydia.

As you read this book, you will find out how different infections vary in their ability to cause symptoms and how, in many people, there may be no symptoms at all. In general, women come off worse than men in this respect, often showing no signs or symptoms of their disease. Nonetheless, there are some symptoms that do give clues and point towards their cause.

## Women's symptoms

*Itching and vaginal discharge* are both addressed in Chapter 3 (p. 26) with candidal infection being the most common cause. Itching around the vulva is also sometimes seen in genital herpes (Chapter 7, p. 83) and genital warts (Chapter 8, p. 92).

*Vaginal odour* is addressed in Chapter 3. A bad smell is usually due to bacterial vaginosis (p. 28), less commonly *Trichomonas vaginalis* (p. 32), and, rarely, a retained tampon (p. 34).

*Dysuria* (stinging or burning when passing urine) in women is most often due to a UTI, see end of this chapter, but is very occasionally seen with chlamydial infection (Chapter 5, p. 59) or gonorrhoea (Chapter 4, p. 47). If the pain comes when urine passes over sore patches outside on the vulva, an 'external' dysuria, then thrush (Chapter 3, p. 26) or rarely herpes (Chapter 7, p. 82) may be the cause in which case there may be difficulty, as well as pain, in passing urine. UTIs may provoke frequency of urination, noticeable particularly at night.

*Unusual vaginal bleeding* will more often be caused by a gynaecological or oral contraceptive-related problem. It is occasionally seen in chlamydial cervicitis (Chapter 5, p. 60).

*Lower abdominal pain (LAP)* can have many causes, from cystitis (inflammation of the bladder) to food poisoning to fibroids, which have no connection with STIs. There can be acute pain associated with chlamydial (Chapter 6, p. 68) or gonococcal (Chapter 4, p. 48) infection and chronic pain associated with adhesions (Chapter 6, p. 73). Non-infectious causes include ectopic pregnancy (Chapter 6, p. 73) and endometriosis (Chapter 6, p. 72).

Pain whilst having sex broadly divides into two sorts. 'Deep' dyspareunia results from the erect penis pushing against sensitive, tender, possibly infected, contents in the pelvis. As with lower abdominal pain (see above) deep pain during intercourse may be due to gonorrhoea or chlamydia and the other causes of LAP. 'Superficial' dyspareunia is when the pain is at the entrance to the vagina or vulva and may be due to infections with thrush or *Trichomonas vaginalis* (Chapter 3, p. 32) or herpes (Chapter 7, p. 82). Poor lubrication may lead to tightness and discomfort (Chapter 3, p. 28).

*Lumps or bumps on the genitalia:* there is a list of the half dozen or so most common lumps and bumps in the section on warts (Chapter 8, p. 93)

*Ulcers on the genitalia* may be caused by trauma, thrush (Chapter 3, p. 26), herpes (Chapter 7, p. 82) or syphilis (Chapter 9, p. 102) and rarely in the UK or USA, the tropical diseases described in Chapter 10.

## Men's symptoms

*Lumps and bumps* are, as in women, addressed in the chapter on warts (Chapter 8, p. 93).

*Dysuria* describes any discomfort when passing water. The term encompasses a 'tingle' and 'pissing broken glass'. Classically a symptom of gonorrhoea (Chapter 4, p. 46) and NSU (Chapter 5, p. 58) it is sometimes found with herpes (Chapter 7, p. 82) *Trichomonas vaginalis* and thrush (Chapter 5, p. 56, and rarely with a UTI, pp 11).

*Urethral discharge* is found with gonorrhoea (Chapter 4, p. 46) and NSU (Chapter 5, p. 52) and rarely with a foreign body (Chapter 5, p. 57). Like dysuria it is sometimes found with herpes (Chapter 5, p. 57) *Trichomonas vaginalis* and thrush (Chapter 5, pp. 56 and 57).

*Ulcers on the genitalia* may be caused by trauma, thrush particularly on the foreskin in uncircumcised men (Chapter 3, p. 26) or herpes (Chapter 7, p. 82) and, rarely in the UK or USA, the tropical diseases described in Chapter 10. Syphilis (Chapter 9, p. 102) is uncommon.

*Redness and/or itching of the glans penis* are classical symptoms of candidal infection (Chapter 3, p. 26) although small flat warts (Chapter 8, p. 93) can give a similar appearance.

*Perianal itching* in both sexes is usually caused by candidal infection Chapter 3, p. 26) although rectal gonorrhea, when there may also be some discharge can cause it (Chapter 4, p. 46). Threadworms (Chapter 10, p. 122) are another cause.

This is not an exhaustive list of possible symptoms and I have purposely not listed any that might be found with HIV infection or AIDS. This is because they are often non-specific, as in a headache or a cough, and unless you reside in an area with a prevalence of 30 or 40 per cent people living with HIV, such symptoms will virtually always be due to something other than acquired immunodeficiency.

## Urinary tract infections (UTIs)

These are addressed here because some UTI symptoms are shared with sexually transmitted infections rather than because cystitis is sexually transmitted, which it isn't. However, symptoms similar to a UTI may be brought on by intercourse, in what used (inaccurately) to be called 'honeymoon cystitis'. When this occurs there is no bacterial infection and the symptoms, of dysuria and frequency are brought on because of poor vulval and vaginal lubrication, with mechanical trauma the outcome. Better lubrication and peeing after sex help with most cases.

Women are more prone to UTIs than men because of the closeness of the urethral opening, just above the vagina, to the anus, and the responsible bacteria are often the same as those found in the intestine. The classical symptoms are dysuria and frequency, particularly at night. There may be blood in the urine, haematuria and an urgent feeling of needing to go *now*.

Recurrent urine infections are not uncommon and are best sorted out by the family physician who should take urine samples (the MSU) to send to the laboratory for identification of the bacteria responsible and the best antibiotics to use. Many people are unwilling to take antibiotics but, with UTIs, particularly if they keep on recurring, failure to eradicate the bacteria may lead to the infection spreading to the kidneys with serious consequences.

Drinking plenty of fluids has always been a good suggestion, but advice to make the urine more alkaline with potassium citrate or sodium citrate, would be more convincing were it not for a number of experts who advocate making the urine more *acidic* as an aid to cure. Cranberry juice is believed by many to ease the symptoms of cystitis but products with added sugar should be avoided.

There is good evidence that completely emptying the bladder accelerates cure rates and can prevent recurrence. It often happens that some urine is left in the bladder after peeing, the so-called 'residual volume'. This is like nectar to the bacteria – they feast, feed and thrive on it. Double micturition, or peeing twice, is the answer. After voiding urine, as usual, stand up and jiggle for thirty seconds or so, sit down and pee again. If more urine appears at this second sitting, you clearly didn't empty the bladder fully the first time. No more proof is needed.

Bizarre as it sounds, double micturition has relieved many women after years of attacks of cystitis and they continue to 'pee twice' as a way of diminishing the chances of further attacks.

## Resources

List of UK Clinics: **www.bashh.org/directory.htm**

List of Australian Clinics: **www.acshp.org.au**

List of US Clinics: **http://www.cdcnpin.org/scripts/locates/LocateOrg.asp?**

# 2 Understanding your results

In this chapter I shall try to make sense of the numbers we come across when reading, talking about, or being tested for, sexually transmitted diseases. I shall try to explain why the investigations you have at your family doctor's or hospital clinic are sometimes unreliable and sometimes downright wrong. You will find figures for how many cases of the different infections were diagnosed in 2003 (the most recent full year available) in the UK and I shall try to explain why these may not be wholly accurate. Before you move rapidly on to the next chapter saying, 'I can't be doing with maths and sums and numbers', let me give you two examples of what I am trying to explain.

*Example 1*: In 2003, over four thousand (4303) new HIV infections in heterosexuals, who were not drug users, were diagnosed in the UK. In the same year, however, less than four hundred (393) heterosexual people (not drug users) actually *caught* HIV in the UK. The figure you will have read in your newspaper will be the 'four thousand' one, coupled with headlines reading 'Heterosexual HIV infection has overtaken homosexual HIV in the UK', giving the impression that this is the extent of HIV actually transmitted in the UK. In fact that year, 3239 of the 4303 heterosexual cases were caught by people when they were living in sub-Saharan Africa whose blood test, however, was performed and then found positive in the UK. In Chapter 11 you will find out how such a flawed system of reporting coloured our views of the HIV epidemic in the 1980s. The 1987 AIDS campaign exhorted us not to 'die of ignorance' while at the same time misleading everybody about the extent of the heterosexual spread in the UK.

*Example 2*: Mrs BB, a 50-year-old married woman from North London went to her GP's surgery to have her routine cervical cytology ('smear test') in January 2005. Because screening for sexually transmitted diseases, in particular chlamydial infection, is so widespread, such a test was taken. In the interests of 'efficiency and cost saving', this chlamydia test incorporated a test for gonorrhoea as well. Mrs BB was telephoned the following week by the practice nurse who told her that she had gonorrhoea and should attend for treatment urgently. The woman's husband was undergoing chemotherapy for prostate cancer at the time and this sudden (and incorrect) diagnosis of a venereal disease put immeasurable strain on their faithful relationship. The gonorrhoea test in Mrs BB's case was a false positive, as it was almost bound to be – see below!

If you are one of the increasingly large number of persons whose partner has tested positive for chlamydial infection, yet your test has turned out negative, you need to know how this is possible. You should not automatically assume that she has been sexually unfaithful (I say 'she' as most of the screening for chlamydia takes place in women).

## Epidemiology

It is common knowledge that chlamydial infection is greatly on the increase – reported cases increased from 53 783 in 1999, to 89 431 in 2003, a jump of 66 per cent. There are reasons why this figure and others should be viewed with a certain scepticism. This 'looking at numbers' is called epidemiology, literally the study of epidemics, and measures, among other things, *incidence*, the number of new cases of HIV, say, that occur this year, and *prevalence*, the total number living with HIV infection each year. The prevalence will include last year's (and all previous years') living cases as well as the new, *incident*, cases from this year.

## Surveillance

Why do we want to count the cases anyway? Well, it is important to be aware of the spread of infectious diseases so that we can try to control them. If the epidemiologists at the Centers for Disease Control in Atlanta hadn't been counting doses of pentamidine (see Chapter 11) in 1981, it might have taken years longer for the AIDS epidemic to have been recognized, many more people would have died, and effective treatments would have been long delayed. Surveillance is the word used for keeping an eye on any change in numbers and is used to detect early evidence of epidemics, be they of food poisoning, this year's 'flu or chlamydial infection.

Testing *some* rather than *all* of a population for a disease is called 'sampling'. By no means all of the UK's residents are tested for HIV every year, but a sample, those giving blood for example, is tested regularly and, if the number of positives in this group of people started to rise, this would give a clue to a possible start of an epidemic. A large anonymous 'rolling' survey of blood taken for other reasons in hospitals continues to monitor levels of HIV infection. Any survey is more valuable if the sample can be shown to be 'representative' of the general population. Thus, surveying injecting drug users in the Bronx for rates of HIV infection would not tell you much about levels of positivity among married farmers in Rochester. The sample tested would not even be representative of the population of New York State.

## Anecdotal evidence

The word anecdote takes on a special meaning for epidemiologists. We all know what an anecdote is – it's a story. For the number crunchers, however, anecdote refers to one particular incident. 'My grandfather smoked sixty cigarettes daily for ninety years and died aged 104 when digging his potato patch.' This is just a story until someone tries to draw conclusions such as 'this shows that smoking is safe' or, less likely, 'digging potato patches is dangerous'. The epidemiologist calls this 'anecdotal evidence'. He would like to see how many people who smoked as heavily lasted sixty, let alone ninety years. 'Well,' you say, 'that's obvious; nobody would be taken in by that, surely?'

At the time of the 'Don't die of ignorance' campaign in the 1980s, a television advertisement showed a young white woman who leant out from the screen and said: 'My name is Mandy, I'm aged twenty-two, I've had two sexual partners and I'm HIV-positive. I am not an actress.' When I first saw the ad, I had just given an Italian injecting drug user the negative result of his HIV test. He was very relieved as he had shared needle and syringe on three occasions with a known HIV-positive patient of ours some six months earlier. Equally truthfully he could have appeared on television with: 'My name is Giovanni, I shared equipment with an HIV-positive drug user six months ago and I'm HIV-negative. I am not an actor.' I am sure that Mandy's story was as true as Giovanni's but the message from these two anecdotes could not be more different. Do not be fooled into thinking an anecdote is equivalent to a representative sample.

## Ascertainment bias

This bit of epidemiological jargon refers to the way in which the true number of events, infections, Roman coins, or whatever, is altered by how hard you go looking for them. One year you come across three denarii in a field next to your house. These are valuable silver coins so you go out and buy a metal detector. Next year, you find fifty. You tell your brother-in-law who brings his metal-detector round and the third year you find two hundred. The numbers have gone up from three to two hundred. Does this mean that more coins have been deposited in the field? No, you've just been looking harder.

Once the importance of chlamydial infection was realized and newer, cheaper, more acceptable ways of making the diagnosis became available, it was possible to screen many more women than before for this infection. Rather like the Roman coins, the more you test, the more you find. There may genuinely be an increase in the *rate* at which women are catching chlamydial infection, last year it was 1000 a week, this year it is 1200, say, but this will be hidden if you are *testing* that many more. Indeed, this extra screening could even be masking a *decrease* in the number of new infections – nobody can tell. What is certainly true is that publicity campaigns which persuade people to attend clinics for testing will raise the apparent number of infections, if only temporarily.

When you next read that there has been a 15, 20 or 30 per cent increase in such and such a sexually transmitted disease, at least pause to reflect on whether this implies a genuine increase in cases.

## How reliable are the tests for infection?

Doctors and other medical staff regularly experience difficulties when trying to explain why certain results may not be reliable. Doctors' inarticulacy may in part be responsible – we are not as well trained in communicating as we are in diagnosing and treating (and I may now be embarking on an exercise that will demonstrate just how inarticulate we are); but a widespread misleading approach to presenting figures and statistics by politicians and salesmen is also to blame. Too much spin makes cynics of us all.

## Laboratory tests

Whenever investigations are undertaken, be they blood tests, urine tests or, as is common in genitourinary medicine clinics, examination of samples using a microscope, there exists some possibility of the result being wrong.

This may simply be bad labelling, such as Mr X's blood being labelled with Mr Y's name. Alternatively, a microscopic appearance may be misinterpreted or missed.

Much of the process of testing in laboratories is now automated. A hundred urine samples are set up in a machine that automatically measures the pH (acidity), the amount of protein, the number and type of cells (white or red blood cells, evidence of infection or bleeding), etc. The machine can go wrong or break down.

The diagnosis of infection is much different from that in early days. At the beginning of the twentieth century, gonorrhoea, say, could be seen using the microscope and a diagnosis made in this way was very likely to be correct. It was also possible to grow (the technical term is *culture*) the gonococcus, the bacterium causing gonorrhoea, in the laboratory. Rather like a green-fingered gardener, the successful laboratory technician takes great care with the culture medium, the 'soil' in which growth takes place and makes sure that all the other factors that influence growth, fertilizer (nutrients), climate (temperature and humidity), environment (oxygen and carbon dioxide content), etc, are perfect for that particular micro-organism.

This sort of 'horticulture' is time-consuming, it takes a good 48 hours for a gonococcus to grow and is expensive in labour and equipment. But after that 48 hours it is possible to say 'this is really very likely to be the bacterium that causes gonorrhoea'. Within a further two days or so, we can say 'it is definitely gonorrhoea' (rather than the meningococcus, a very close relative that causes meningitis and can sometimes be found in the genitalia) and, further, 'it is resistant to the following antibiotics' (the bad news) 'but treatable with these' (the good news).

This sort of test, laboratory culture, has a very high *specificity*. That is to say, if it says it's gonorrhoea, gonorrhoea it is. Or, of one hundred positive gonorrhoea results, one hundred will actually be gonorrhoea. Assuming the growing conditions are correct, the test will also have a very high *sensitivity*. This means that, if you had one hundred people who genuinely have gonorrhoea, the test will detect all one hundred of them.

Let us deal with sensitivity and specificity, in more detail for they are crucial to the understanding of why today's tests may give the wrong answer.

## Sensitivity and specificity

These two measurements of how good and useful a test can be, answer two different questions.

The first is: 'If the test is positive, is it truly positive? You say I've got gonorrhoea. Are you sure?' How *specific* is the test? So the first question addresses the specificity of a test. Will there be false positives?

The second is: 'If I have got gonorrhoea, will your test be positive? Will my condition be picked up by your test?' How sensitive is your test? The second question addresses the question of sensitivity. Will there be false negatives?

I could stand at the entrance to my clinic and tell everybody that they had gonorrhoea. As a test for gonorrhoea it would be a pretty poor one in that it would generate a large number of false *positives*. But, and this is of interest, it would treat every single case of gonorrhoea that walked into the clinic. It would not miss any cases. It would be a very sensitive test.

Or, I could stand at the entrance to my clinic and tell everybody that they did not have gonorrhoea. Because almost all the people who attend have *not* got gonorrhoea, this would be quite a specific test. It would be right in almost all the cases. But it would miss the few positives.

The relative importance of sensitivity or specificity can vary considerably in different circumstances. Let's look at examples of how these two concepts might assume different importance:

*Sensitivity*: I have been unfaithful to my wife. I had sex with a woman without using a condom last week. My wife is returning from abroad shortly and I need to be sure that I won't infect her with gonorrhoea when she gets back. I need a highly sensitive test. If I have caught gonorrhoea, I need it to be diagnosed and treated. A false negative would be disastrous but a false positive wouldn't matter too much as I can live with being unnecessarily treated on this occasion. If the test gave a false negative, I would pass on gonorrhoea to my wife and that would be the end of my marriage. The test for gonorrhoea needs to be sensitive.

*Specificity*: I have been accused of giving gonorrhoea to our au pair girl. Two weekends ago she came home with a boyfriend who spent the night. My wife has forbidden the au pair to have boyfriends to stay but was away that weekend. The au pair has been diagnosed with gonorrhoea and, rather than admit that the boyfriend stayed over, she claims it was me who gave her gonorrhoea. I have not slept with the au pair and I do not have gonorrhoea. A false negative would not matter but a false positive would be a disaster. If a false positive result arrived, my wife would believe the au pair and that would be the end of my marriage. The test for gonorrhoea needs to be specific.

Fair enough, so all we need is a test that is sensitive and specific, that shouldn't be too difficult, should it? Well, it is. Problems arise because the sorts of tests we use nowadays do not make use of the old-fashioned 'horticultural' methods of growing gonorrhoea (or chlamydia) which, like planting a cabbage seed, give you a definitive answer when it has grown. You cannot mistake a cabbage for a carrot. Or the meningococcus for the gonococcus. Some of today's tests (nucleic acid amplification tests, or NAATs) detect part of the bacterium's nucleic acid rather than detecting, or growing, the whole organism. The tests tend to be highly sensitive – if the infection is there, they will find it. However, this sensitivity is at the expense of specificity. There will be some false positives.

## What numbers affect the usefulness of a test?

We saw earlier how epidemiologists describe, for example, the number of new cases of gonorrhoea per hundred thousand people per year (in London, in women aged fifty it is about four). They also find it useful to describe the number of false positive tests per hundred thousand tests. For the test used on Mrs BB (at the beginning of this chapter), it is about 370 false positives per hundred thousand. You can see now why any positive from testing Mrs BB for gonorrhoea was virtually certain to be a false positive.

Even though the false positive rate is very low, less than one, at 0.37 per cent, when it is used to test a population of people who have an even lower prevalence of disease, most of the positives will be false. As the screening programmes are rolled out yet further into the community, so the number of false positives becomes greater when compared with the true positives.

The NAATs tests used for chlamydia screening have the same strengths and weaknesses as the gonorrhoea tests. They are sensitive; they will detect infection if it is present but they will also generate a significant number of false positives. These will, perhaps, be more noticeable when they turn up in an unlikely scenario like Mrs BB's above, but what if Mrs BB had been aged 22 and recently engaged? There would have been no questioning her positive chlamydia result with all its ramifications. One expert from the chlamydia screening programme in the UK recently suggested that the 10 per cent prevalence of chlamydia in young women, a figure generally bandied about to demonstrate the parlous state of affairs, is almost certainly nearer 5 per cent in the general population.

## The equivocal result

Reports from a laboratory that a test is 'equivocal' are an inevitable result of using investigations, such as some for chlamydia, which do not culture a particular bacterium (or virus) but identify a part rather than the whole of it. Many tests use differences in colour to determine whether or not they are positive, with, for example, a change from transparent to red denoting that the organism is present. Transparent is manifestly different from red: nobody could mistake one for the other. A machine is often used to 'read' the colour of a test and its range might be from 0 (absolutely transparent) to 50 (dark red). So far, no problem. But supposing the test result turns out pink. Well, if it is a dark pink (the machine reads 45), one might say that it is very likely to be positive. If, on the other hand, it is barely pink at all (the machine reads 5) most would agree that it's a negative.

What if the result is 25, however? Or 39, or 10, or 16? This is where an arbitrary decision must be taken by those making or using the test as to where the cut-off point between negative and positive should lie; and here we have come full circle back to sensitivity and specificity. If you choose the cut-off point at, say, 5 (barely pink at all), you will have a very sensitive test – it will pick up the very slightest of infections. But, and it is a very big 'but', you will have a large number of false positives. Mrs BB and her husband will not be pleased. If, however, you make the cut-off point 48 (pretty damned red), say, you will have a very specific test – your positives will all be real, genuine, cast-iron positives – but, and it is an equally big 'but', this test will not be sensitive enough to catch all the positives. Some, perhaps early infections, or those in which the sample was not big enough, will actually be positive but the test will not detect them. You will have false negatives.

So how do the decision-makers handle this dilemma? There are two possible solutions. The first is to set an (inevitably) arbitrary level, say 25 – all results above 25 are positive and all below are negative. This approach will give a number of both false positives and false negatives but it shouldn't matter too much as most results will be red or transparent, 50 or 0. And, indeed, it won't matter, unless you happen to be one of those wrongly diagnosed positive or whose infection has been missed. The second solution is to pick a range of readings, say 15 to 35 (slightly pink to quite pink), which you term 'equivocal' and on which you postpone a decision until you have repeated the test on a second sample.

This has been a necessarily simple explanation of how equivocal results come about. The tests may be compromised by other factors – there are substances found in urine that alter the sensitivity or specificity of an investigation, as may physical factors such as temperature or the time since a sample was taken. If the laboratory is in doubt, it needs to test a further sample. Their polite way of asking for a second sample is to call the first result 'equivocal'.

## National figures for sexually transmitted infections

Cases of sexually transmitted infections, including HIV, are collected in the UK by the Communicable Disease Surveillance Centre, which is part of the Health Protection Agency (HPA). Scotland returns its own figures and those quoted for the UK include English, Welsh and Northern Irish cases. As I write, numbers are available to the end of 2003.

The greatest increase, referred to earlier in this chapter, is in reported chlamydial infections which increased from 53 783 to 89 431 in the five years between 1999 and 2003. Gonorrhoea increased from 15 974 to 24 157 over the same period and syphilis from 215 to 1580. Genital herpes, at 16 581 to 17 932, and genital warts, at 66 439 to 70 665, both showed comparatively small increases. There remains a question mark over the chlamydia figures because of ascertainment bias but the other numbers probably reflect reality with reasonable accuracy.

Total new HIV cases in the UK increased from 3095 to 6928 per year between 1999 and 2003. Imported cases, largely from Africa, made up the large majority of the heterosexually acquired numbers.

## The situation worldwide

Geographical variations in HIV infection are dealt with in detail in Chapter 11 but the numbers of cases in different regions vary just as the predominant modes of transmission differ.

As of the end of 2004, an estimated 25.4 million persons were living with HIV infection in sub-Saharan Africa. This gives an adult prevalence of 7.4 per cent. The next highest prevalence is in the Caribbean at 2.3 per cent although the numbers infected are much fewer at 440 000. Asia provides the highest number of infected individuals, after Africa, at 8.2 million although the prevalence of infection is lower at 0.4 per cent. However, this low prevalence serves to highlight the awful potential of a full-blown HIV epidemic in this part of the world – were the prevalence the same as sub-Saharan Africa's, at 7.4 per cent, there would be 151.7 million persons infected in Asia at the present time.

In the USA the majority of HIV positives are gay men who have suffered increasing levels of STIs in recent years. In Los Angeles and San Francisco, syphilis has been seen to go up six-fold in a three-year period. The total number of HIV positive persons has not altered significantly in the past ten years, at around one million.

Eastern Europe, including Central Asia, has an overall HIV prevalence of 0.8 per cent with a total of 1.4 million cases. The Russian Federation accounts for 70 per cent of all cases in the region, at slightly less than one million.

Australia, New Zealand, the Middle East and North Africa have, between them prevalences less than 0.2 per cent – their potential for increasing numbers is discussed in Chapter 11.

## Resources

For UK figures see: www.hpa.org.uk

# 3  Vulval and vaginal problems

Although this is a book devoted mainly to sexually transmitted infections, there are a number of other genital problems that affect women and may mimic conditions that are sexually transmitted or which may be brought on by intercourse. Vulvo-vaginal thrush is a case in point: we frequently see patients who are convinced that they have acquired some frightful condition from a recent sexual partner because of soreness that came on during or soon after sex. Particularly if this was a first episode of sex after a period of abstinence, this onset of symptoms may simply reflect a pre-existing candidal infection that was aggravated by the rubbing and friction of sex. Likewise, there are a number of skin conditions that may make sex uncomfortable or sore. How is one to know that these are not, say, herpes?

Thus, the conditions dealt with in this chapter come under the two broad headings of vaginal discharge and vulval problems, which, coincidentally and in that order, make up the two most frequent reasons for women attending GUM clinics.

## Vaginal discharge

The majority of discharges seen in a specialist clinic are not sexually transmitted although some of them may be related to intercourse. Each woman tends to be aware of her own 'normal' vaginal discharge and also aware that this may vary over the menstrual cycle, for example, becoming a little thicker towards the beginning of the period. Others regularly have a little spotting of blood in mid-cycle coinciding with ovulation.

## Is there a normal amount of vaginal discharge?

One might as well ask if there is a normal height for a grown woman. One of the medical registrars working in our department at St Thomas' in the

1980s, Maggie Godley, tried to find out what was the normal amount of vaginal discharge. She asked some of her patients whether they thought their discharge was heavy or light in quantity, or normal. She also recorded *her own* impression of quantity while performing the clinical examination. She then asked each patient to take away an ordinary tampon which was inserted and left in the vagina for one day. This was brought back to the clinic in a plastic bag and weighed.

Not surprisingly, there was a large variation in the amount of discharge picked up by the tampon in 24 hours, but what was odd was that there seemed to be no correlation between what the patients thought was a heavy discharge and the weight of the used tampon, nor was there any relation between that and what the doctor had observed. In short, there seems to be a wide variation in 'normal' vaginal discharge and neither the owner of the vagina nor a professional observer seem able to agree consistently on whether there is too much, too little or just the right amount. Message? Women know their own bodies very well and what may appear normal to an examining doctor or nurse may not be normal for the woman concerned. If you notice an alteration in your discharge, it probably has altered!

There is an expected, and normal, increase in vaginal discharge at puberty and in women taking the oral contraceptive, particularly if it contains oestrogen. Most women notice a decrease in their normal discharge when they reach the menopause.

## Should my discharge smell?

Ask any pubertal schoolboy and he will tell you that women smell 'down there'. Indeed, it seems an almost universal belief. I am sure that mothers don't tell their sons at an early age of this supposed female characteristic. Yet the myth persists, reinforced by silly 'jokes': in New York, in the window of a Broadway T-shirt shop where the picture/logo/quote of your choice is printed on to a shirt, 'If it smells of fish, eat it'.

For whatever reason, it is a received belief that there is likely to be a nasty odour associated with the female generative organs. This, of course, is not so. In the groin (of both sexes) there are apocrine glands, as there are in the armpits, which produce secretions with an odour. This is a normal, healthy, human smell and has nothing to do with the nasty smells alluded to above. There are infections of the vagina that are responsible for unpleasant odours, *Trichomonas vaginalis* and bacterial vaginosis, but neither of them is natural or 'normal'. If there is a 'fishy' smell, then something should be done about it – see the following sections.

# The normal vagina

The vagina, after the stomach with its hydrochloric acid, is probably the most acid part of the body. It has a pH (see below) of less than 4.5 which makes it an unattractive environment for most bacteria, although, sadly, not *Candida albicans*. The local inhabitants, lactobacilli, the 'good' bacteria, not only thrive in, and depend on, acid surroundings but produce hydrogen peroxide which stops other bacteria surviving and reproducing.

As we shall see, anything that alters this vaginal ecosystem and, in particular, anything that kills the lactobacilli or makes it less hospitable for them is likely to result in a higher (less acid) pH and to let in other, often smelly, bacteria. These other bacteria are present in all adult females on the perineum but would normally be kept at bay by the acid and hydrogen peroxide.

# Vulvo-vaginal candidiasis (thrush)

The most common infection found in the vagina, and on the nearby skin, is thrush, or candida. Figures vary but probably two-thirds of all adults have candida in their intestines as a commensal, that is, an organism that co-exists without harming the host or being harmed by it. Although it resides in the gut, it is excreted along with the stools at defecation and both men and women are equally likely to develop infection around the bottom, peri-anal candida. Women, however, are disadvantaged by their anatomy and the proximity of the anus to the areas in question explains their propensity for developing vulval and vaginal candidal infection.

*Candida albicans*, although the most common, is only one of several sorts of *Candida* that can be found in humans with *Candida glabrata* being the other vaginal pathogen.

# Why do women get thrush?

In many, if not most cases, there does not seem to be any particular reason for thrush developing. The anatomical reasons given above map out its easy route from intestine to vulva or vagina but why infection happens in some rather than others is not clear. There are, however, some pre-disposing factors that do greatly increase the likelihood of developing thrush. People with diabetes or who have higher than normal levels of steroids (either because of self-production, as in the rare Cushing's disease, or because steroids have been prescribed for another medical condition) often suffer. In addition, those who have been taking antibiotics that kill off the healthy bacteria in the vagina are prone to candidal infection. People whose immune (defence) system is not functioning efficiently are also more prone to developing thrush.

## What are the signs and symptoms?

Candida does not always cause symptoms but, when it does, it makes its presence known in two ways. First, by an accumulation of infected debris (in women, this shows as a white vaginal discharge) and, second, by causing itching and irritation, often with some soreness. The textbooks attribute a 'classical' appearance to the discharge, 'like curds or cottage cheese', but, in most cases, the vaginal discharge is thin and may be very slight. Some women describe a yeasty smell.

The itching is due to candida's powerful ability to provoke what is, in effect, an allergic reaction. When a body is sensitized to thrush, a very small infection can provoke itching that may be quite out of proportion to the amount of *Candida* that is present. Occasionally, such an intense reaction is set up that the vulva swells up (become oedematous) and becomes sore, if not painful. The vagina itself does not itch, except at its entrance, the introitus. The skin of the lips (labia) may also be infected, as may the skin between the vagina and the anus (the perineum) and the anus itself. Fissures may occur on the skin, which are partly sore and partly itchy. These tiny, thin, reddish lines, up to a centimetre in length and with a waxy appearance of the surrounding skin, make the diagnosis of thrush likely.

A woman with vulvo-vaginal thrush may, thus, have itching/soreness alone, discharge alone, itching/soreness and discharge, or no symptoms at all.

In men, the same conditions apply, although it is unusual to accumulate much discharge and this occurs only in men who have not been circumcised. However, the itching can be just as intense as in women and primarily affects the glans penis (the tip of the penis) and the foreskin, if present. The glans may become inflamed and raw, with tiny, flat, red marks on it (a condition doctors call posthitis). Occasionally, the foreskin will swell as a result of candidal infection but, like the oedema of the vulva in women, this is uncommon. Some men who have been sensitized to thrush can diagnose the infection in their female partner because they get a feeling of hotness and itch on the glans penis within a few seconds of starting to have sexual intercourse.

## What tests might I have?

In the majority of thrush cases, the combination of vulval itching and vaginal discharge makes the diagnosis obvious to the woman concerned and her medical or nurse adviser. As treatments are available without prescription from a chemist, many women prefer to buy their own over-the-counter medication. Similarly, going to the GP with these symptoms is likely to lead to a prescription for antifungal treatment without the need for laboratory tests to confirm the diagnosis. If the symptoms keep recurring or do not seem to respond to the treatment, then there are advantages in knowing that *Candida* is truly responsible for them and that the treatment prescribed is the correct one.

A definite diagnosis of thrush is made either when the fungus is seen using a microscope or when a sample of vaginal discharge or from a scraping of infected skin is cultured in the microbiology laboratory. The advantage of using the laboratory is that the fungus can be accurately identified and examined in case it is resistant to the commonly used anti-fungal treatments. This resistance testing is not undertaken routinely in laboratories as it is expensive and the large majority of thrush organisms are sensitive to the standard treatments.

## What treatments are available?

There are two basic sorts of treatment available: those that are applied directly to the infected parts, such as pessaries or creams to be inserted into the vagina, used in conjunction with creams or gels that are rubbed onto the outside skin; and tablets to be taken orally. Both can be bought direct from a chemist shop. There is a huge and lucrative market for these antifungal agents and much drug-company money is spent promoting the particular advantages of one product over another. Other than in excep-tional circumstances, it is very difficult to show that one product has a better cure rate than another and the major considerations should be how much it costs and how acceptable the product is to the user. Most GUM clinics prefer to use pessaries and creams rather than oral tablets for vulvo-vaginal thrush, although the tablet treatment is obviously easier to take.

Successful treatment depends on eliminating the fungus from both the vagina and the skin of the vulva, perineum and around the anus, and many failures of treatment stem from the lack of proper treatment to this surrounding skin. If there have been symptoms of itching or soreness, it is crucial to apply the antifungal cream for an adequate time. Fungal infections do not disappear overnight. I usually suggest using the cream (sparingly – a centimetre rather than an inch from the tube) twice daily for at least a fortnight, making sure to cover all the skin from the clitoris down to the area surrounding the anus and rubbing it in well (and washing your hands afterwards). Threadworms may be a cause of perianal itching.

Antifungal cream is also prescribed for candidal infection in men. It is rubbed on to the end of the penis and foreskin but it is equally important to remember that your sexual partner almost certainly also has thrush, whether or not there are symptoms, and the balanitis is likely to recur until they are treated.

Some antifungal creams are combined with a weak steroid, often 1% hydrocortisone (HC), and these may be beneficial when there is a great deal of soreness and itching. However, this combination should be used sparingly.

## Are there any complications of the condition?

Physical complications are not an important feature of candidal infection but it can cause problems with sexual intercourse. A woman with thrush may experience soreness and even pain when having sex and this may lead to a disruptive vicious circle that can compromise a happy sex life. For a woman to enjoy sex, she needs to be in the mood, relaxed and naturally lubricated. A woman's lubrication, like a man's erection or even salivation, is not under conscious control – one cannot just decide to lubricate, salivate or become erect! Worry, fear or anxiety can each block these natural functions. If a woman has experienced discomfort during sex because of thrush, she may well be anxious that it will happen again when next she tries. This nervousness stops relaxation and lubrication and so the cycle repeats itself. The vicious circle can be broken when the thrush is properly treated and, perhaps, some artificial lubrication is used to help return function to normal.

Most women with thrush will be cured following a single treatment although there is always a possibility of fresh infection, particularly after taking antibiotics. In some women the candidal infection seems to keep on recurring and this may be due to reinfection of the vulva and vagina from the surrounding skin, especially that between the vagina and anus. If thrush seems difficult to eradicate it is worth going to the GUM clinic where the staff are used to dealing with this problem.

## Bacterial (anaerobic) vaginosis (BV)

Bacterial vaginosis, sometimes known as anaerobic vaginosis (AV), is a common cause of vaginal discharge and genital odour and, like thrush, is not a sexually transmitted infection.

## Why do some women get BV and not others?

Bacterial vaginosis occurs when the inside of the vagina, the vaginal environment, is disturbed with a change in its acidity. The normal, healthy vagina is more acidic than other parts of the body and contains hydrogen peroxide, a powerful antiseptic. Bacteria called lactobacilli, useful germs, produce the acid and hydrogen peroxide, which discourage other germs from surviving or taking over. The 'bad' germs consist of *Gardnerella vaginalis* (not to be confused with gonorrhoea) and a hotchpotch of anaerobic bacteria, which are bacteria that can survive without oxygen. It is these anaerobes that are responsible for the odour in BV.

You may hear doctors talking about pH, which is a method of measuring acidity. Confusingly, the lower the pH, the more acid and the higher the pH, the less acid there is. Neutral, neither acid nor alkaline, measures 7 on the pH scale. The healthy vagina has a pH lower than 4.5. If this reading becomes higher, the lactobacilli stop thriving and there is an opportunity for the other bacteria to replace them. This is what happens in bacterial vaginosis.

These other bacteria are found in healthy women but in such small numbers that they do not cause any problems or symptoms. So what makes the vagina less acid? The most commonly quoted causes are soaps, shampoos and bath gels. Indeed, most bath additives, including bubble baths, can be responsible. This is because these sorts of products tend to be alkaline, the opposite of acid. Douching (using a shower head or spray to wash out the vagina) is associated with frequent recurrences of BV.

What is less well-known is that even just letting bath water into the vagina may also make it less acid and encourage the development of BV. This is because plain ordinary water will kill lactobacilli just as efficiently as soap or shampoo. Many women will lie in the bath, part their legs and 'swish' or 'swill' water into their vagina to clean it out. In some women water just gets into the vagina without any help. If, when you stand up from a bath, water comes out of the vagina, there is a good chance that you are damaging those vital lactobacilli. It is counter-intuitive but 'the more you wash, the more you smell'.

Bacterial vaginosis is a condition that only affects women. Men do not have an equivalent infection to BV. Some studies have shown the presence of the germs that cause BV in the male urethra but this is not a constant finding nor is there evidence that the germs in men will cause BV in an otherwise healthy woman.

## What are the symptoms of BV?

Although, as with thrush, there may be no symptoms from BV, the usual complaints are of an increase and alteration in vaginal discharge coupled with an unpleasant smell, typically described as 'fishy'. Some women are acutely aware of this odour and believe that everyone near them will smell it. This is virtually never the case.

The condition is called vaginosis because there is no significant inflammation of the vagina or vulva. Words ending in '-osis' simply mean 'condition of', as opposed to those ending in '-itis', which means inflammation. Thrush causes a vaginitis, BV a vaginosis. This means that BV does not cause itching, irritation or soreness.

One of the features of BV is its inconstancy. The symptoms may wax and wane, may have a relation to the stage of the menstrual cycle and may be associated with sexual intercourse. This variability may cause problems when trying to establish the diagnosis if the condition happens to be on the wane at the time the woman is examined.

## What are the tests for BV?

A changed discharge and nasty smell points towards the diagnosis. While an absolutely definite diagnosis could be made by taking a sample of discharge and culturing it in the laboratory for the bacteria that are responsible, this is time-consuming, expensive and, in practice, unnecessary.

When the facilities are available (as they are in all GUM clinics) the bacteria can be readily seen using a microscope, the pH can be measured using a disposable strip of special pH paper and a 'sniff' test can be performed. This entails mixing a little of the vaginal discharge with potassium hydroxide, an alkaline, and noticing the particular smell that is given off, a mixture of chemicals called aromatic amines. These have self-explanatory names like 'putrescine' or 'cadaverine'. Some women with BV particularly notice the smell after sexual intercourse, when the man has ejaculated in the vagina. The ejaculate is itself alkaline and releases the smelly chemicals in the same way as potassium hydroxide.

## Treatment of BV

Highly effective antibiotics are available for the treatment of BV but it is important to remember the predisposing causes mentioned above and avoid all bath additives. In addition, don't wash your hair in the bath; don't douche and don't let water into the vagina. With regard to that last bit of advice, some women have controlled their recurrent BV by 'putting a plug in it', that is, placing two cotton wool balls (or using a tampon) at the entrance to the vagina before getting in the bath (and remembering to remove them afterwards).

The main treatment has for a long time been an antibiotic called metronidazole which is usually prescribed for five or seven days or, occasionally, given once in a large dose. A newer antibiotic, tinidazole, can also be taken as a one-off.

Another antibiotic, clindamycin, can be used as a 2% cream that is inserted in the vagina or taken orally as tablets for a week. Both the antibiotics have a high cure rate, particularly if any predisposing factors are dealt with. There is no evidence that treating the male partners of those with BV makes any difference to the cure rate or the risk of recurrence.

Metronidazole reacts very unpleasantly with alcohol in a number of people and must be avoided while on treatment. Metronidazole used to be avoided in the first three months of pregnancy but recent studies have shown it to be completely safe.

Recurrent BV can be a real problem for some women and various different regimens of treatment are being tried for these difficult cases. Use of a metronidazole vaginal gel twice weekly for a period of four to six months or oral treatment for three days just before and just after menstruation look to hold some promise. There is, however, and slightly sadly, no evidence that use of live yoghurt or addition of bacteria, *Lactobacillus acidophilus*, makes any difference at all.

## Are there any complications of the condition?

There is currently a debate about the importance, or otherwise, of BV during pregnancy. Some studies have suggested that for women who have had a premature baby or have lost a baby in mid-pregnancy, the presence of BV may increase the likelihood of the same thing happening again and that they should, therefore, be treated when next pregnant if BV recurs. Other trials have failed to demonstrate that such treatment makes any difference. The consensus is that until we can be absolutely certain one way or the other, it is probably safer to treat BV in pregnancy in those who have previously had problems.

There is good evidence to suggest that several of the organisms found in BV may also be responsible for part of the damage occurring in some cases of pelvic inflammatory disease (PID) and metronidazole is often added to the other antibiotics used in treatment of PID. Likewise, some experts suggest treating women with BV who are having a surgical procedure such as termination of pregnancy.

Bacterial vaginosis, with the possible exceptions of pregnancy and pelvic infection mentioned above, is a harmless condition. Some women seem to get frequent recurrences but strict avoidance of douching and bath additives, shampoos etc., in the bath water usually stops these. It can be helpful to use condoms for a period to prevent the alkaline ejaculate raising the pH of the vagina.

## *Trichomonas vaginalis* (TV)

Trichomoniasis is a sexually transmitted condition caused by *Trichomonas vaginalis*, a protozoon (a single-celled organism like an amoeba) that may produce nasty vaginal symptoms in women but often goes unnoticed in men who are infected. In the past it was frequently found in combination with gonorrhoea but, in the UK, such a pairing is no longer that common.

## What are the signs and symptoms?

The symptoms in women are similar to those of bacterial vaginosis – that is, vaginal discharge with an unpleasant smell. Anaerobic bacteria, as described above, are almost invariably found along with trichomonas and the pH is higher than normal (less acid) with a loss of lactobacilli, those bacteria that are so useful in keeping the vagina healthy. These anaerobes, along with a distinctive contribution from the trichomonads, are responsible for any nasty odour.

The vaginal discharge may be quite profuse but, in contrast to BV, TV can be associated with a marked inflammation. BV is a vagin*osis* (i.e. a condition of), whereas trichomonas causes a vagin*itis* (i.e. an inflammation of).

The inflammation of the vaginal wall can be severe. Additionally, the vulva may become inflamed to the extent of causing pain and soreness on passing urine (dysuria). The discomfort is due to warm urine passing over the inflamed skin on the outside. This 'external' dysuria should be distinguished from the discomfort found on passing urine in cystitis (bladder infection), which is 'internal'. External dysuria can be associated with very bad thrush or an attack of genital herpes. Sometimes, there is so much discharge in TV that it leaks on to the inner surface of the upper thighs, giving a sore, reddened area known as a 'tide-mark'. Sex can be very uncomfortable when it is severe. That said, some women may be infected with *Trichomonas vaginalis* for years without noticing any symptoms at all.

In men, infection with TV may also cause nothing in the way of symptoms. Alternatively, it may cause a urethritis (inflammation of the urethra – the tube that takes urine to the outside world), giving mild discomfort on passing urine and a slight urethral discharge, or sometimes no symptoms at all.

## How is the diagnosis made?

The distinctive nasty smell and the discharge or inflamed vulva and vagina may give a clue but the definitive diagnosis is made by identifying the amoeba-like protozoon using a microscope.

A small amount of vaginal discharge is mixed with dilute salt solution (saline) and, when examined microscopically, reveals characteristic pear-shaped objects moving around, propelled by their flagellae, which are extensions of the cell wall and act like oars. Examination of the vaginal discharge suspended in saline is a routine test in all GUM clinics, although the finding of TV is rare. It is also possible to grow (culture) the parasite in the laboratory but, as the diagnosis is made so readily by microscope, the time and expense of culture does not justify its use.

A third, and potentially misleading, diagnostic tool is cervical cytology: the smear test. Although this test is designed to detect pre-cancer or cancer of the cervix, it can also show cells that indicate infection with herpes simplex or wart virus. If *Trichomonas vaginalis* is present, it can also be seen, but (and an important 'but') there may be other cells that look like TV and this may lead to a mistaken diagnosis. When TV is genuinely present, it will be readily identified at the GUM clinic.

Diagnosis of TV in men is unsatisfactory. Although the parasite is undoubtedly present in a man's urethra, looking for it in a urethral sample suspended in saline only identifies it in perhaps 10 per cent of men who are known contacts of a woman with TV. We know that it is present in a much higher number of contacts than this, but the ways of proving it would be so unpleasant for the man (massage of the prostate gland or massage of the penis with a metal rod in the urethra, see Chapter 5) that most men who are contacts are given treatment anyway.

## What is the treatment?

The mainstay of treatment is the same drug that is used for BV, metronidazole. It is used over five or seven days, or given as a single large dose. Metronidazole reacts badly with alcohol in a number of people and it should be avoided when taking this drug. Although there are other related compounds that have a similar therapeutic effect, there is no other treatment that has been shown to work as well. In the days before metronidazole had been discovered, a woman with TV might carry the parasite throughout her life. In those days, treatment with pessaries (vaginal tablets) made from arsenic compounds could be effective but they ran the risk of causing severe inflammation of the vagina. Sometimes *Trichomonas vaginalis* becomes resistant to metronidazole and the old-fashioned treatment with acetarsol pessaries is a reasonable alternative. I have yet to see a bad reaction to this treatment.

# Are there any complications of the condition?

Under normal circumstances, the answer is no. However, there is some evidence that TV, like BV, is associated with premature birth or small babies; as with BV, the jury is still out. In a small number of cases where the mother gives birth while she has the infection, her female child can be infected as she passes through the birth canal.

The vagina returns to full health following treatment but it is important to remember that the infection may return unless the male partner is also treated, which he should be, whether or not TV is found in him.

# Other infections causing discharge

It has been noted that both gonorrhoea and chlamydial infection are associated with an increase in vaginal discharge. I am sure that this is true but unfortunately in neither infection is there any characteristic of the discharge to give a clue to patient or doctor as to the diagnosis. Gynaecology textbooks describe the discharge of gonorrhoea as 'yellow or green' whereas STI textbooks go for 'purulent or blood-stained'. When we made a note of the discharge, during a study of gonorrhoea, the most common description was 'white'. If a primary attack of herpes affects the cervix there can be a profuse muco-purulent discharge that appears to be vaginal unless one examines the cervix itself.

# Foreign bodies

Foreign bodies (see Chapter 5 for these in men) are found in the vagina just as they are found in the urethra and rectum and are an uncommon cause of vaginal discharge. The intra-uterine contraceptive device (IUCD) is a foreign body (it is *in* the body but not *of* the body) and is associated with excess discharge in some women. The tampon is another foreign body and one which, if forgotten and left behind, is responsible for a particularly foul, persistent discharge which once diagnosed, however, is easy to treat.

Young children are prone to insert objects into their ears and nose as well as their mouth but with the dawn of sexual awakening, a second phase of insertion is seen in males and females, at first in an exploratory fashion and then as an aid to masturbation. Hence the finding of vibrators or beer bottles in the rectum. However, it is usually easier to retrieve a foreign body from the vagina than the rectum.

## Case history

Bridget T, a 14-year-old schoolgirl, put a hairpin into her vagina and couldn't get it out again. She was too embarrassed to tell her parents and, as she felt no pain and developed no problems, she ignored it and then forgot about it. A few years later, and unusually for these days, she went to see her GP for family planning advice, prior to sleeping with her boyfriend (it is more usual to have sex first and then think about contraception). She had had a bit of vaginal discharge and so the GP, before prescribing the pill, took some vaginal swabs and examined her internally.

He was measurably surprised to see two sharp prongs projecting down into the vagina from just beside the cervix. In the intervening years, the hair-pin had perforated the vaginal wall, turned through 180° and lodged near the cervix. After a minor operation Miss T was able to start off her relation-ship properly protected against unwanted pregnancy and posing no threat of grievous injury to her unsuspecting boyfriend.

# Vulval problems

Women often complain of itching discomfort or pain on the vulva and, in most cases, the cause is simple and the treatment is easy. By far the most common cause is candidal infection.

## Case history

Mrs SB had intractable vulval itching. This had started a year or so previously, following three bouts of cystitis which had each been thoroughly treated with antibiotics. She had used over-the-counter pessaries from her local chemist but, after a week when these had made no difference, she visited her GP. The locum doctor took a sample from her vagina (a high-vaginal swab, or HVS) to send to the laboratory and prescribed more pessaries. When she returned two weeks later, no better, she was told that the swab test was neg-ative and that perhaps it had not been thrush, after all. She was prescribed a weak steroid cream, 1% hydrocortisone, which eased her symptoms for a short time but three weeks later her symptoms had returned. During the next six months she attended a private clinic four times and on each occasion an HVS was taken and more antifungal vaginal treatment prescribed.

None of this worked and she was desperate when she returned finally to her local practice. When she explained her problems, the GP examined her and, for the first time in nearly twelve months, took a sample from her vulva. This came back from the laboratory showing a good growth of *Candida* species. Mrs SB had to use the antifungal cream for three weeks before her itching and soreness had gone.

It is a strange fact of life that gynaecologists and GUM physicians are so used to taking samples from inside the vagina that even when the answer is given directly to them by the patient, 'I'm sore and itchy on my labia', it is the vagina rather than the vulva that is tested.

## Skin conditions

Almost any condition that affects the skin elsewhere, from contact dermatitis to psoriasis, can involve the vulva but there are a small number of conditions that occur more frequently than others. There are three 'lichens' that affect the vulva, each different but each treated, at least initially, with strong steroid ointments.

If one itches, one scratches. If one scratches on a daily (or more usually nightly) basis, the skin becomes thickened and damaged, a condition called lichen simplex or neurodermatitis. It is often provoked by stress and emotional upsets. Lichen planus is characterized by small slightly raised violaceous spots, which can leave the skin pigmented after healing. These usually cause little or no trouble but in some cases, the areas of skin become raw and painful, so-called erosions, which also occur in the mouth. Finally lichen sclerosus, which sometimes runs in families and can affect young children, is responsible for soreness and cracked skin. If they have been present for a very long time, both lichen sclerosus and lichen planus can progress to skin cancer but this is rare and easily picked up by the skin specialist.

Cancer of the vulva is associated with HPV infection just like carcinoma of the cervix (see Chapter 8). Vulval intraepithelial neoplasia (VIN), is HPV-associated in more than 90 per cent of cases and is pre-cancerous in the same way as cervical intraepithelial neoplasia (CIN) on the cervix. Imiquimod, although it can produce a lot of local soreness, has a beneficial effect on a majority of those treated. Imiquimod is a local immune modulator and seems to be effective in other pre-malignant skin conditions including Paget's disease of the vulva.

It is important not to forget the role of irritants in the production of vulval signs and symptoms. Urine, sweat, semen or faeces can all provoke an irritation as can sanitary towels, panty liners or incontinence pads. Some treatments, like podophylline or imiquimod for warts, can cause symptoms and even ordinary soap may be responsible for a nasty reaction. Contact dermatitis, a local allergy, will need a specialist dermatologist to unravel.

# Vulvodynia

This is a catch-all symptom defined by the International Society for the Study of Vulvovaginal Disease, the ISSVD, as chronic discomfort or pain in the vulva which may be 'burning, stinging, irritation or rawness' when there is no infectious or skin disease to account for it. Generalized vulvodynia involves the entire vulva including the clitoris and pubic area, or it may affect different areas at different times.

The vestibule is the oval-shaped area of skin between the labia, between the clitoris and the perineum. Women with vulval vestibulitis syndrome (VVS) have discomfort limited to when, or immediately after, that part of the vulva is touched. Sexual intercourse, insertion of a tampon or a speculum, indeed anything that exerts pressure on the vestibule brings on the characteristic burning sensation. Women with VVS not only have their daily routine disrupted – it may be uncomfortable just sitting – but many find it difficult or impossible to have sex. Clinical depression is a not uncommon feature with feelings of low self-esteem.

In the early days there was thought to be an association between VVS and human papillomavirus infection but it now seems that HPV is found no more and no less frequently than in the unaffected population. Biopsies have suggested that there may be a local alteration of the immune response, possibly due to recurrent candidal infection. In some women with cyclic vulvovaginitis, which comes and goes, often depending on the stage of the menstrual cycle, long-term treatment with oral antifungals has been successful.

Other treatments for VVS include strong steroid ointment which, if used for a month or so, gives marked improvement in perhaps 30 per cent of women. Amytriptyline, an antidepressant, works consistently in most of these chronic vulval conditions but it is important not to give the impression that the symptoms are simply psychological – these are real physical conditions with a medical, organic basis. One of the difficulties that arises is sensitization of the vulval skin to all the various products that are applied so regularly. Certainly, if long-term recurrent candidal infection is suspected, it may be better to use oral antifungal agents rather than topical creams or ointments.

Finally, post-menopausal women may suffer from the unhappily labelled 'senile' atrophy which describes the ageing of the vulval and vaginal skin when there is less oestrogen circulating. Oestrogen has an important role to play in promoting storage of glycogen which is involved in the production of lactic acid and maintenance of the low pH in the healthy vagina. Five years after the menopause there is a 30 per cent reduction in skin glycogen. Senile atrophy is a relatively easy diagnosis to make which is readily treated with topical oestrogen cream.

One of the most successful, and innovative, approaches to vulval pain has come from the development of a multidisciplinary team to look after different aspects of the patient's problem. The doctor, psychotherapist, physiotherapist and dietician see the sufferer, in that order, and empower the patient by involving her in decisions about the way in which her condition is to be managed. Many women have only discussed their problem with a GP and few with their partner. In one study, the very giving of a diagnosis, the labelling, was found to give significant relief in 85 per cent of women. The recognition that theirs was a genuine condition which carried no stigma put them well on their way to recovery.

## Resources

Vulval Pain Society (VPS): **www.vul-pain.dircon.co.uk**

National Vulvodynia Association: **www.nva.org**

**www.bashh.org/guidelines.htm**

# 4 Gonorrhoea

## Historical aspects

It was in the second century AD that Galen invented the word 'gonorrhoea' (from the Greek: $\gamma o \nu \eta$ = semen and $\rho \varepsilon \iota \nu$ = to flow) but the disease had already been recognized for many centuries by Greek philosophers and sages such as Hippocrates, Plato and Aristotle. A passage in the Old Testament, 'When any man hath a running issue out of his flesh, because of his issue he is unclean' probably refers to gonorrhoea. Other excerpts from Leviticus, Chapter 15, include: 'And when he that hath an issue is cleansed of his issue; then he shall number to himself seven days for his cleansing, and wash his clothes, and bathe his flesh in running water, and shall be clean', which might be an early reference to the infectious period, and 'he that sitteth on anything whereon he sat that hath the issue shall wash his clothes, and bathe himself in water, and be unclean until the even', suggesting that the myth of the lavatory seat as a source of infection pre-dates the invention of the flush toilet by at least two thousand years.

The proper microbiological name for the bacterium that causes gonorrhoea is *Neisseria gonorrhoeae*, crediting Albert Neisser with its identification in 1879. In fact, a Professor Hallier had noticed the characteristic micro-organisms using a microscope, in the pus cells of gonococcal discharge, some seven years earlier. Had the learned professor had been a little more ambitious, we might now be referring to the gonococcus as *Hallieria gonorrhoeae*.

What Hallier and Neisser had found were tiny kidney-shaped bacteria actually inside white cells, part of the body's defence against infection, arranged in pairs known as diplococci (two cocci). These are comparatively easy to see, using a strong magnification of one thousand-fold, when stained with a dyeing process called Gram's stain. They show up with a pink colour (Gram-negative) giving the last of the three criteria for a microscopic diagnosis of gonorrhoea, which are: Gram-negative, intra-cellular, diplococci (GNID). There are several other bacteria similar to the gonococcus which belong to the same family, the *Neisseriae*, the most important of which is *Neisseria meningitidis*, a cause of severe bacterial meningitis. Very rarely *N. meningitidis* can cause a urethritis, proctitis or cervicitis and, if looked for, GNID may confusingly be seen using the microscope. *N. meningitidis* is a normal inhabitant of many people's throats and fellatio may explain its presence in the urethra.

## How is it caught?

Gonorrhoea is almost exclusively acquired sexually – by penetrative vaginal or rectal intercourse, fellatio or cunnilingus. Nobody knows exactly how infectious gonorrhoea is but the penis is the most efficient transmitter of gonorrhoea. Thus a man with urethral gonorrhoea is more likely to pass on the infection than is a woman with cervical, or a man or a woman with rectal or pharyngeal infection. My own opinion, and it is only an opinion, is that a man with gonorrhoea will have an upwards of 95 per cent chance of passing it on to a woman with whom he has vaginal sex. The figure for a woman passing it on to a man might be between 60 per cent and 80 per cent. The risk will obviously increase the more times intercourse occurs.

Nobody knows how long a time it takes for somebody who has caught gonorrhoea to become infectious to someone else but there are case reports of onward transmission within an hour or two of acquisition. If wishing to exclude gonorrhoea in someone who has been at risk, particularly a woman, I prefer to wait at least three days to allow the organism, if present, to multiply enough to ease detection.

Can it be caught from a lavatory seat? Well, it is possible, but it would be extremely difficult and this excuse would need to be a man's rather than a woman's. This is because the gonococcus dies very rapidly away from the warmth and moisture of a human being. It is just possible (although in 35 years of practice, I have never seen or heard of such a case) that a man's penis could lodge a little discharge on a seat or the inside of a lavatory bowl, when sitting, and that a second man's penis could come into contact with the discharge before the organism had perished. The gonococcus cannot infect ordinary skin surfaces, needing mucous membrane or internal tissue. It is therefore unlikely that a woman could either infect a lavatory seat or bring an infectable part of her anatomy in contact with one.

## Case history

Dr Harald M was asked to see a Scandinavian sea captain who had just come into harbour with his catch of North Sea cod. He complained of a urethral discharge that had come on some seven days into his two week fishing trip. The Captain vigorously denied any extra-marital contacts in the previous year or more and nearly came to blows with the doctor when asked about any possible homosexual contacts on his all-male ship. 'Certainly not!' was the emphatic answer. The only possible explanation was that he had caught it from his wife and, after giving the antibiotics, the Captain was asked to bring in his spouse soon for examination.

Two hours later, Dr M was consulted by the First Mate from the same fishing vessel who was complaining of a urethral discharge that had come on two days into their recent fishing trip. He likewise vigorously denied any homosexual activity but did admit to a casual fling with a young lady he had met in a bar three days before his ship had set sail originally. Further probing (this had to be done carefully because Dr M could not break the Captain's confidence) revealed that the First Mate owned a full-size blow-up plastic female doll with holes in all the right places. 'Does anyone else use it?' prompted the answer 'No' – except that, on this last trip, the Captain had visited his cabin and, seeing the manikin, had exercised his Captain's prerogative and borrowed the doll. When the Captain returned to the clinic the following day, his discharge now gone, he admitted to having used a plastic doll for sexual relief and (having been reassured by Dr M that no secrets had been divulged) was able to return home, his honour and marriage intact.

The above true story was published by a reputable medical journal (Dr M was subsequently awarded the 'alternative Nobel prize' by Harvard University) and demonstrates the possibility of infection by contact with another's discharge.

There are two important exceptions to the normal sexual mode of transmission of gonorrhoea – newborn infants and pre-pubertal girls. If a mother is suffering from a gonococcal infection of the cervix (the most commonly infected site) when she gives birth by vaginal delivery, there is a good chance that the baby will become infected. The most common site will be the baby's eyes giving ophthalmia neonatorum (see page 67 for chlamydial infection of a newborn's eyes) which, in olden times, was the commonest cause of childhood blindness. It is an increasingly rare complication in the West today. The eyes, throat and vulva may also be infected and it is therefore wise to give oral antibiotics as well as topical ones when gonorrhoea is diagnosed.

The second non-sexual mode of transmission is via inanimate objects such as towels or flannels. Before girls reach the age of puberty, the vulva and vagina have a different hormonal and glycogen content which makes them, unlike the case in adults, a good breeding ground for the gonococcus. Nowadays everyone is much more aware of child sexual abuse and, while this possibility must never be discounted, it should not be assumed to be the case, particularly in the very young child. Before the antibiotic era there were several reports of outbreaks of gonococcal vulvo-vaginitis on wards or in dormitories where the serial abuse of twenty or thirty young girls was rather unlikely compared to, say, the infected rectal thermometer that had been used consecutively on all the inmates.

## Case history

Professor Natalie V, a specialist microbiologist, was transporting clinical samples from several nearby clinics to her laboratory while trying to look after her 18-month daughter, strapped in a child seat in the back of the car. She had a collection of agar plates which are plastic dishes containing nutrients for the various bacteria one might be trying to grow. Samples are inoculated onto these plates for subsequent culture in a laboratory. 'Chocolate' agar contains no chocolate but is so named because one of its ingredients, heated blood, has a Hershey-like brown colour.

When she reached her laboratory, the Professor was horrified to find that her baby had reached over and was quietly munching her way through the jelly-like contents of one of the agar plates that had been recently collected from a local STI clinic. There was enough of the inoculated sample left to put into an incubator in the laboratory and 48 hours later, there was a tell-tale growth of colonies of gonococci on the plate. A throat swab from her daughter, taken at the same time, grew an identical organism – probably the youngest verified case of oro-pharyngeal gonorrhoea ever – but innocently acquired.

Mouth-to-mouth transmission between adults is theoretically possible but it must remain an unlikely and rare route. Whereas we frequently see throat infection in women or gay men who perform fellatio, perhaps because the penis is in direct contact with the back of the throat, it is highly unusual to see such cases in men who have practised oral sex, cunnilingus, on an infected female partner. This is because the man's mouth is in contact with an area not infected in its own right, the clitoris and vulva. Just like gonorrhoea caught from a lavatory seat, I have never come across a case of direct mouth-to-mouth transmission but that may be because throat infection tends to give no symptoms, it is the one site where spontaneous elimination of the organism occurs, and, finally, clinics do not routinely screen people's throats for gonorrhoea unless there is evidence of the infection elsewhere.

## Are there many cases today?

The number of reported cases of gonorrhoea has gone up and down like a roller-coaster since figures began to be reliably collected after the First World War. In the UK there was a noticeable peak in 1946 followed by a precipitate drop to the mid-1950s (see Fig. 4.1). This fall was ascribed to the increasing availability of penicillin but, I am sure, was quite independent of this. You will note a similar, if smaller, drop in 1919 when there were no antibiotics of any sort and, indeed, the early (swinging) 1960s heralded not only a rapidly increasing gonorrhoea epidemic but a coincidental rapidly increasing selection of new effective antibiotics. Both peaks probably reflected a number of cases in returning servicemen (the accepted explanation) but, more importantly, ascertainment bias (see Chapter 2) – there were more important things to do during the war years than count the number of cases of gonorrhoea.

Gonorrhoea reached its peak incidence in the mid-1970s, with over 60 000 cases in England, compared with some 11 780 cases in 1994. The decrease has been attributed to changing sexual practices as a result of the fear of AIDS but, in truth, the decline had started several years before the HIV epidemic became apparent. Reported cases have started to rise since 1995.

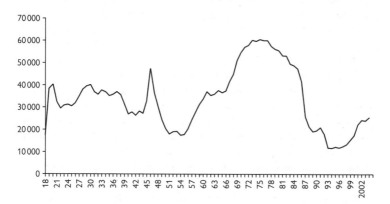

**Figure 4.1** UK Gonorrhoea figures 1918–2004

# Who catches it?

There are remarkable and consistent differences in the number of cases of gonorrhoea between different ethnic groups and sexual orientations. In the UK, the large majority (over 90 per cent) of gonorrhoea cases among men who have sex with men (MSM) occurs in Caucasians while an equally disparate figure appears for gonorrhoea in heterosexual men. Several studies, after controlling for age and social deprivation, demonstrate a real difference in rates of infection between persons of African and Afro-Caribbean origin and between both these groups and Caucasian populations. Similar findings have been published in the USA regarding higher rates of infection in those of African-American and Hispanic origin.

In Chapters 11 and 12 we explore the differences in incidence of HIV infection in various parts of the world as well as the role of other STIs in determining the likely transmission rates of HIV. Gonorrhoea not only acts as an 'accelerator' to the transmission of HIV but is probably the best marker of HIV risk. Gonorrhoea, unlike so many other STIs, is readily and easily diagnosed and, in men at least, produces instantly recognizable symptoms and signs.

To catch gonorrhoea or HIV, you need to have had unprotected sex. Catching the one denotes immediate risk of the other.

# How is gonorrhoea diagnosed?

The usual sites infected are the urethra, throat and rectum in men, and cervix, urethra, rectum and throat in women. Rectal gonorrhoea in the male is usually the result of insertive rectal intercourse although infection can be passed on by vibrators or digital insertion. In 40 per cent of women with gonorrhoea, the infection is found in the rectum and there is no need for rectal intercourse to have taken place (although, as with MSM, it may have done). The simple action of gravity combined with eversion of the anal mucosa during intercourse allows infected secretions to come into contact with anal tissue. The cervix is the most commonly infected site (90 per cent) in women, followed by the urethra (75 per cent), rectum (40 per cent) and throat (anything from 3 to 15 per cent). In about 5 per cent of cases each, the rectum or urethra will be the only site from which the gonococcus can be identified. So, if one is trying to exclude gonorrhoea, it is crucial to sample all four sites.

If a diagnosis of gonorrhoea is to be made, samples must be taken for testing from all the possible infection sites listed above. Microscopy, the examination of a stained sample using a high magnification, is the mainstay of diagnosis in a GUM clinic and has the great advantage that, if positive, a diagnosis can be made on the spot. This works well for men who, if there is a significant urethral discharge, will have the diagnosis made in well over 95 per cent of cases. GNID are easy to see in men with penile gonorrhoea. Infected women, by contrast, are less likely to yield up their diagnosis. Even when cervical, urethral and rectal samples are stained and examined, less than 50 per cent will be found to reveal the diagnosis with microscopy. The same sort of figure applies to samples from the male rectum. For all its lack of sensitivity, microscopy does offer the chance of an instant diagnosis and most clinics still practise it as a routine.

Growing the gonococcus in the laboratory (see Chapter 2, page 17) remains the mainstay of diagnosis and allows the possibility of examining the organism's sensitivity to different antibiotics. Because microscopy is insensitive for samples from women, culture assumes a more important role than in men. The culture medium (the agar plate gobbled up by Professor V's daughter) contains meat extract, the 'chocolate' heated blood, and various antibiotics and antifungal agents to prevent other bacteria or funguses from growing as well.

The final tests for gonorrhoea (blood tests are discounted – none has yet to give even half-reasonable results) are the 'indirect' tests, nucleic acid amplification tests (NAATs). These are dealt with in some detail in Chapter 2 when the problems associated with their lack of specificity are highlighted. However, these tests are not all bad. They appear to be highly sensitive – if the gonococcus is present, they will identify it and they may turn out to have particular value in sites that are less easy to sample effectively, such as the throat and rectum. But, as emphasized, problems arise when they are used as screening tests in very low-prevalence populations.

## What are the signs and symptoms?

In men, gonorrhoea as a cause of urethral symptoms has been eclipsed by chlamydia and non-specific urethritis, which, between them, are also much more important in terms of their complications in women. However, the symptoms of gonorrhoea, particularly the discharge, are certainly more florid than those of *Chlamydia trachomatis* and one interesting aspect of gonococcal infection is the way in which it has changed over the years as a result of the introduction of antibiotic treatment.

The incubation period, the time between infection and the development of symptoms, has progressively lengthened since records were first made in the 1930s. In that pre-war era, men noticed something wrong within two or three days, on average. By the 1990s, the average time had increased to over eight days. Coincidentally, the severity of the dysuria, the pain on passing urine, seemed to have diminished significantly. There is no generally accepted measure for pain, the way there is for, say, weight (in pounds or kilos), or height (in feet or metres) but there are two indications that there has been a genuine change in symptoms.

The first is of an anecdotal nature, in that we rarely see patients complaining of the really severe discomfort, so often mentioned in the old textbooks. The old descriptions of gonorrhoea talked of dysuria as: 'Pissing broken glass', 'like razor blades' and 'a red-hot poker in the pipe' (the French referred to it as *chaudepisse* – hot piss), whereas, these days, someone with gonorrhoea may only mention, in passing, a slight 'tingle'. Indeed, 50 per cent of those attending our clinic in London with gonorrhoea do not mention any discomfort at all.

The second indication of a less severe symptom is the longer time it takes today for someone with gonorrhoea to attend a clinic once they have developed symptoms. In the 1930s the average time was under three days whereas now it is nearer six days. It could be that the pre-war sense of urgency, driven by extreme discomfort, is missing today. There is no indication, however, that the discharge has altered significantly.

Why then should the incubation period have lengthened and the pain diminished? These changes are real ones and, I believe, reflect adaptations by the gonococcus to changes in its environment. Before antibiotics, there would not have been any pressures on the bacterium to alter in any way. However, once adverse pressure arrived in the form of effective and lethal antibiotics, there would be a selective advantage to those strains of the gonococcus that produced fewer symptoms, later. They would have a greater chance of being passed on to another person before the penicillin destroyed them. The one-celled organism divides every five minutes and one would almost be able to watch adaptive evolution taking place before one's eyes.

The discharge of acute gonorrhoea, however, remains as profuse as ever. Saying that, it should be remembered that the discharge – off-white and staining the underwear – will initially be no more than a slight bit of mucus and takes a day or two to develop into full-blown pus, of which there may be a great deal. Clinic workers recognize the 'tissue-paper' sign – when a man attends with a piece of tissue paper on the inside of his underwear, the diagnosis is gonorrhoea, until proved otherwise.

Gonorrhoea of the rectum tends to produce no symptoms at all in more than 80 per cent of men (or women) with the infection. A few will notice some pus on their faeces and others may complain of a little dampness or itching around the anus but most will be blissfully unaware of their infection.

Infection of the throat is not associated with any particular symptoms although it seems that those, men or women, who practice oro-genital sex are more prone to sore throats than others.

## Case history

Gladys H was a 37-year-old separated sweet-shop owner in a south coast holiday resort and was named as a contact by a young man with gonorrhoea. She was upset by this accusation and said that this young man was the only person she had slept with, and only once, since her husband had left her some ten months previously. When she was examined, the vagina and cervix looked quite healthy, and microscopy and culture from cervix and urethra were both negative for the gonococcus on two occasions. She failed to return for follow-up.

The incident was forgotten until the young man returned five months later with another attack of gonorrhoea. He said he had once again had sex with Mrs H and was certain that she was the source of his infection. With some reluctance she agreed to have a further examination but the doctor this time included the rectum, in addition to the cervix, urethra and throat, as a site of possible infection. Both the stained microscope slide and subsequent culture were positive for the gonococcus. Although both she and her paramour denied rectal intercourse, this site was probably the source of the infection, which had been presumably acquired from her husband over a year previously.

With regard to infection in women, the gonococcus is a microbiological master of male chauvinism, not only being difficult to diagnose using the microscope but also producing little help by way of symptoms or signs to lead physician or patient towards the diagnosis. In women, there may be no helpful symptoms at all in perhaps 50 per cent of cases. Some women mention an alteration in vaginal discharge but this has no particular characteristics. Discomfort on passing urine, said to be common years ago, is no longer a major feature. A woman may therefore have to rely (like Gladys H) on the development of symptoms in her partner to alert her to the possibility of gonorrhoea.

As 75 per cent of women with gonorrhoea have the infection in the urethra, one might have expected that urethral discharge, as in men, would be a notable sign, if not symptom. However, the female urethra is much, much shorter than the male's and thus has less length of tissue to become inflamed and to produce discharge. The urethral opening is hidden between the folds of the labia and even if a woman were to examine herself, the natural moistness of this part of the body will tend to mask any contribution from the urethra. Perhaps one in eight women will complain of dysuria but, when one considers what a frequent symptom this is in young women, it is a poor indication of infection.

Other symptoms that might give clues as to the possibility of gonococcal infection in the woman, arise late and are mostly produced as a result of complications, such as infection spreading to the fallopian tubes.

## What are the complications of gonorrhoea?

The complications of gonorrhoea in women are, in almost all cases, the same as those associated with chlamydial infection, as detailed in Chapter 6. Local infection of glands around the vulva can cause a bartholinitis, painful swelling on the labia, or skenitis, a similar condition next to the urethra. These are both comparative rarities in the West today.

Spread of infection inwards can give rise to endometritis, followed by involvement of the fallopian tubes, salpingitis and into the pelvis to give pelvic peritonitis. It does not seem possible to distinguish between the signs or symptoms associated with chlamydial salpingitis and those found in gonococcal salpingitis. Of course, both infections may be found together in the same patient. Either infection, once it has spread internally, may lead to problems with fertility including the implantation of a fertilized ovum in the wrong place, an ectopic pregnancy.

Lower abdominal pain is a persisting problem with pelvic infection as may be 'deep dyspareunia', discomfort felt during intercourse when the penis is inserted to its full length. This also occurs sometimes in perfectly healthy women because of contact between the penis and the ovaries. A woman's ovaries are just as exquisitely sensitive as a man's testicles and would hurt just as much if they were kicked. They are normally protected within the bony pelvis but there are certain occasions during sex when penetration is deeper, when the woman is on top, for example, and the erect penis will bang the ovary, particularly if it hangs a little lower in the pelvis. This is known as 'anvil' syndrome after the metal block on which a smith might fashion a horseshoe.

Spread of infection internally can, as with *Chlamydia trachomatis*, give rise to Fitzhugh-Curtis syndrome, a condition in which the lining outside the liver becomes inflamed, a peri-hepatitis. Whether caused by chlamydial or gonococcal infection, this is hard to recognize as the patient presents to the doctor with pain under the right ribs which can even cause some problems in the lungs. It is difficult to reconcile with an infection originally caught through sex.

The important exception, unique to gonorrhoea, is spread of infection via the blood stream to almost anywhere else in the body. In practice this means spread to the skin, where small pustules appear which may have a little bleeding in them, and the joints which are inflamed but rarely severely damaged. This is in contrast to the pre-antibiotic era when infection of a joint with gonorrhoea would usually lead to enough damage to leave the joint crippled beyond repair. Other 'old-fashioned' complications included hepatitis, meningitis (mimicking its cousin, the meningococcus) and even endocarditis, in which the valves of the heart become infected. That this was a life-threatening complication is illustrated by the title of a scientific report dating from the 1930s entitled: 'Gonococcal endocarditis – a report of twelve cases, *with ten post-mortem examinations*' (my italics). The only reports of this condition since the Second World War have come from the USA although there was one unpublished case in London in the 1980s.

Because they are much more often symptomatic with their gonorrhoea, men are less likely to develop its blood-borne complications but they may develop infection in one of the various glands that contribute their secretions in the genital area. There are small openings inside the urethra called Littré's glands and various others including Cowper's, Tyson's and the prostate gland. Any of these may become infected with swelling pain and discharge of pus. The gonococcus can also, like chlamydia, cause an epididymo-orchitis.

## How is it treated?

In 1937, the *Journal of the American Medical Association* reported the first successful treatment of gonorrhoea using a sulphonamide, M&B 693, and there was unqualified rejoicing from patients and doctors alike. The treatments that were superseded had included urethral irrigation, in which a strong antiseptic solution was run into the urethra under high pressure to 'wash out' the germs, while progression of the infection was monitored by regular urethroscopy, the passing of a rigid metal tube with telescope attached, into the urethra to obtain direct visual confirmation of resolution of the urethritis. It was around this time that penicillin was being evaluated and developed in Oxford and London so that, when cases of gonorrhoea inexplicably stopped responding to the sulpha drug, there was an alternative readily available. It is said that, during the war, penicillin was reserved for soldiers with venereal disease rather than those with, say gangrene, because the VD patients could be returned to the front more readily.

This loss of efficacy of the sulphonamides was the first example of development of bacterial resistance which has dogged the use of antibiotics ever since. *Neisseria gonorrhoeae*, along with *Staphylococcus aureus* (the 'SA' in MRSA), is one of the micro-organisms that has most obviously taken advantage of an ability to alter its metabolism to make it impervious to these drugs.

The susceptibility of *Neisseria gonorrhoeae* to antibiotics differs throughout the world in direct relation to the extent of their misuse in different countries. Where antibiotics are readily available without prescription, over the counter or in a market stall, there will be ample opportunity for the gonococcus to gradually develop its reduced sensitivity to these agents. Thus, *Neisseria gonorrhoeae* is more likely to be resistant to penicillin in parts of the Far East or Africa than in the UK.

In terms of treatment options, we remain ahead of gonorrhoea, but only just. A group of antibiotics called the cephalosporins remain effective throughout the world but there is little in reserve if resistance should develop to those. As I write (mid-2005), the UK recommendations for treatment of gonorrhoea have just been changed from a penicillin or a quinolone to one of the cephalosporins because of increasing resistance to both the first two.

## Resources

www.bashh.org/guidelines.htm

# 5 Non-specific genital infection

Non-specific genital infection (NSGI) is a general, catch-all term for a number of genital conditions affecting men and women that are characterized by the difficulty of making a precise diagnosis at the time of first attendance, hence the 'non-specific' element of the name. Non-specific urethritis (NSU) is the condition from which the others follow, not because it affects men rather than women (which it does), but because NSU is the most likely of the family of non-specific conditions to cause symptoms – it is the man who will notice something wrong first.

In men, NSU can be caused by a variety of germs but, in the majority of cases, no micro-organism can be identified; in most cases the cause, at the end of the day, is truly non-specific. The most important single cause of non-specific infection is *Chlamydia trachomatis* but, as with any of the other infectious or non-infectious causes, there are no readily available means for confirming such a diagnosis on the spot.

## What is NSU?

We have discussed what 'non-specific' means. Urethritis is an '-itis', or inflammation, of the urethra (as in laryngitis, an '-itis' of the larynx or appendicitis, an '-itis' of the appendix). There are many, many factors that may cause an inflammation in the urethra, some due to micro-organisms, like gonorrhoea, chlamydial infection, or herpes, and some resulting from irritants, like excess alcohol intake, foreign bodies (18 inches of 1 mm diameter pink plastic tubing in the penis – another story), or very spicy foods. This inflammation provokes a natural response from the urethra in the form of local production of white cells, one of the body's natural defence mechanisms, called polymorpho-nuclear leucocytes (PMLs), or 'pus cells' in common parlance. When pus comes out of a boil it is made up of bacteria and these pus cells. It is unusual to see frank pus in urethritis unless gonorrhoea is present; more often the discharge will be muco-purulent, pus cells mixed with mucus, or simply mucoid and clear to the naked eye. The mucoid discharge may, however, contain a significant number of PMLs and the pus cells may even be present when there is no obvious discharge at all.

## How is a diagnosis of NSU made?

Here we come to the first of two major problems with NSU (the other being the slightness of the symptoms). With most infections, there is a test which, if positive, confirms that the infection is present. This might be a blood test that finds antibodies to the infectious agent. Alternatively, the bacterium, fungus or virus can be seen using a microscope or be cultured in the laboratory. While it is true that *Chlamydia trachomatis* can be positively identified, most cases of NSU are not chlamydial in origin. There is no test for the majority of NSU that can confirm the presence of infection.

The first indication of NSU will come from the symptoms (see below) or perhaps a history of exposure to possible infection. If infection or inflammation is to be confirmed or excluded, we need to know whether there is a urethritis: are there pus cells present? Under normal circumstances there should be no pus cells within the urethra. There are two ways of getting at the inside of the urethra: a recently passed urine sample can be centrifuged (spun rapidly so that any solid matter, including cells, is reduced to a pellet) or a 'smear' taken with a small loop or swab passed directly into the urethra. Either way, the sample obtained is smeared on a microscope slide, stained to show up the cells and bacteria in colour, and examined with a high-power lens, usually enlarging the image one thousand-fold. In my department at St Thomas' Hospital, the centrifuge was junked several years ago for 'health and safety' reasons.

For diagnosis using a microscope, perhaps ten or twelve areas of the stained slide, known as fields, are examined and, if textbooks and learned papers in learned journals are to be believed, the pus cells are counted in each. The number of pus cells per high-power field (PCs per HPF) is then averaged to arrive at a magic figure, which indicates the degree or severity of the urethritis. Thus, you would expect to, and indeed usually do, see more pus cells in a sample from a man with a purulent discharge than one with a slight mucoid discharge briefly, first thing in the morning. The average number of pus cells is then placed into a category to give a semi-numerical scale, for example: 0 (none), $+/-$ $(1-9)$, $+$ $(10-19)$, $++$ $(20-29)$ and $+++$ ($\geq30$). In real life, the process is different. The pitfalls of such a system are enumerated in Chapter 2, but suffice it to say, what appears to be a scientific and exact system for evaluating urethritis is nothing of the sort and may be responsible for faulty diagnoses.

This pseudo-scientific system for evaluating not just the presence but the degree of severity of NSU is unreliable. The pus cells may be due to an infection and, in many first-time cases, probably are. But they may not be.

Of course, when the stained urethral sample is examined, one may find evidence of gonorrhoea (see Chapter 4) when the bacterium, the gono-coccus, is visible under the microscope. This then becomes a diagnosis of gonococcal urethritis. As gonorrhoea is effectively the only infection that can be reliably and consistently confirmed in these circumstances, all other cases of urethritis diagnosed in this way are non-gonococcal urethritis (NGU). 'NGU' is an alternative label for 'NSU' and is preferred to 'NSU' by purists, in spite of which, most clinicians and patients still refer to the condition as NSU.

So, gonorrhoea is absent and pus cells are present. Does that mean that an infection is present? Well, a heavy drinking session may result in enough alcohol being passed out in the urine that it inflames the urethra resulting in a 'chemical' urethritis. When these pus cells are examined microscopically, they are no different from those found when infection is present. Some have suggested that hot spices, as in a vindaloo, may give a urethritis. In other cases, where it is inconceivable that a sexually trans-mitted condition could be present, no explanation for the inflammation can be found.

Other tests will be taken at the time of NSU diagnosis and treatment, the most important of which will be a test for chlamydial infection. If that comes back positive, the urethritis is no longer non-specific but chlamydial.

## What are the *possible* causes of NSU?

Over the past fifty years a number of different organisms appeared and were championed as the magical 'organism X' which would explain NSU and its frequent recurrences. I mention a number of *possible* causes in some detail as, in various parts of the world, they are regarded as definitely responsible for disease (pathogenic) and can be vigorously, and expen-sively, sought and treated. If either of the first two below has been diag-nosed and treated in Milan, Marseille or Mill Spring, Missouri (population 252), do not panic, just don't send any more good money after bad.

When I joined the specialty in 1971, we had just eliminated *Mycoplasma hominis* from our list of causes of NSU. This small bacterium had been found in the secretions of men with NSU and not in those without. In fact, 70 per cent of men with NSU were found to have *M. hominis* but its position as organism X was comparatively short-lived when a fatal flaw was found in the original work that had suggested it as a pathogen.

This trial was very convincing until it emerged that the men without *M. hominis* or NSU were not strictly comparable with those who were infected. The crucial difference lay in an important behavioural characteristic of the 'uninfected' group. They were not sexually active. When a group who *were* sexually active, but didn't have NSU, were used as a control for comparison, they were found to have infection with *M. hominis* just as frequently. *M. hominis* was, and is, sexually transmitted, but so are babies. Neither is a sexually transmitted disease. In several European countries *M. hominis* is regarded as a pathogen in the urethra but the evidence simply does not back up this belief.

Before we leave *M. hominis* it should be said that this organism has been implicated in some cases of acute kidney infection or pyelonephritis, and is thought to be involved in a few cases of pelvic infection in women. So it certainly is capable of causing disease. Just not NSU.

Next to emerge, as a minuscule answer to our prayers for the causative organism, was 'T'-strain mycoplasma ('T' is for tiny), *Ureaplasma urealyticum*. This little bug earned its credibility when two eminent researching venereologists, serious and scientific both, having first ascertained that each was completely free from any possible infectious cause for NSU and indeed from the condition itself, inoculated each others' urethras with *U. urealyticum*. Both developed a rip-roaring urethritis that lasted for several weeks and included generalized 'flu-like symptoms. Having subjected themselves to this ordeal, they became understandably zealous proponents of *U. urealyticum* as the long-awaited missing cause. It is possible that *U. urealyticum* is, or can be, a pathogen in a small number of cases but, as with *M. hominis*, it is so often found in normal folk without infection, that its role in NSU must finally be consigned to a very minor one.

A short but illustrative digression. The above story is an example of what I have called the 'toothpaste theory' of science. If for the active ingredient of a scientific experiment, one can substitute toothpaste, without materially affecting the outcome of the experiment, one should sprinkle the experiment and its conclusions with question marks or at least take on board a healthy helping of scepticism. At the beginning of the AIDS epidemic in the early 1980s, much pressure was brought to bear on scientists who were working with potential cures for HIV infection, to try this or that magic compound because, when the compound was added to the human immunodeficiency virus growing in cell-culture in a test-tube, it was shown to kill the virus. However, toothpaste added to HIV in a test-tube kills the virus, and toothpaste, for all its other acknowledged attributes, is not a cure for AIDS. The fact that toothpaste causes a urethritis does not prove that toothpaste is *not* the cause of NSU but it certainly does not prove that it is. The same argument holds for *U. urealyticum*.

There will be some anguish from my peers that I have included *Mycoplasma genitalium* as the third micro-organism in this section of the chapter for, like *M. hominis* and *U. urealyticum* before it, there are avid supporters for this most recent of causes of NSU, in Europe, the UK and the USA. This latest in the *Mycoplasma* family was first identified in 1989 and has subsequently been shown to be present in cases of NSU. As an object of scientific investigation it suffers from two important drawbacks. It takes up to four weeks to grow in a laboratory (by contrast, you can grow the gonococcus or chlamydia in 48 hours) and, at present, there is no readily available test that is sensitive and specific enough to make the diagnosis in a laboratory setting. So, we are currently unable to prove or disprove its importance.

## What are the *accepted* causes of NSU?

The most important cause of NSU is *Chlamydia trachomatis*. Chlamydia, as I shall (incorrectly) call it for simplicity's sake, is a bacterium, but a highly adapted one. It has a lifestyle more akin to that of a virus, in that it cannot survive outside a living cell. This means that, if you wish to grow it in the laboratory, you cannot simply take a sample from an infected site and plonk it onto or into a growth medium and wait for it to multiply as one would with other bacteria, like MRSA, for example. It has to be kept alive in a transport medium on its journey to the laboratory where it is then placed in contact with living cells that it can infect in order to replicate.

Cell culture is a difficult, time-consuming, expensive and unreliable method of growing an organism and is nowadays confined to research laboratories and medico-legal cases. Culture of chlamydia is, of course, a way of demonstrating its presence with no possibility of doubt (assuming the sample is actually from the person whose number is on the bottle) but, as it is not a sensitive method (you may only grow it in 70 per cent of actual cases), it is routinely replaced by tests which purport to identify bits or pieces of *Chlamydia trachomatis*, or parts of its DNA.

The first of this new, non-culture, ways of identifying chlamydial infection were called ELISA or EIA tests. They were said to have a higher sensitivity than culture (they found more of the real cases) but had certain problems with specificity (more false positives). These sorts of tests are being phased out but are still, for reasons of financial economy, to be found in some non-hospital settings.

The most modern tests now in use are variations on nucleic acid amplification tests (NAATs). These appear to have very high sensitivity (very few false negatives) but a small problem with specificity (false positives) that can become a large problem if the tests are used indiscriminately for everybody. The problems of false positives in populations with low disease prevalence are referred to in more detail in Chapter 2.

Blood tests detecting antibodies in chlamydial infection are of little, if any, use in individual patients although they may be of use in large population studies.

For all the potential problems with modern methods of diagnosis, nobody questions that chlamydia *is* the important cause of NSU. Lots of major studies involving tens of thousands of patients in the 1970s and 1980s, when culture was the only sensible and readily available diagnostic tool, demonstrated that when chlamydial infection was present in the urethra, a urethritis ensued. It is true that in many cases of NSU it was not possible to find chlamydia but it had never been claimed that it was the *only* cause. Chlamydial infection was also found in the partners of men with chlamydial urethritis and in the fallopian tubes of those who went on to develop infection there, salpingitis.

*Trichomonas vaginalis* (see Chapter 3), TV for short, is a one-celled animal, like an amoeba, which is sexually transmitted. It also happens to be particularly hard to find in the male although the urethritis that it causes is self-evident. Figures vary but most studies that have looked at male sexual partners of women with TV have only managed to find it in about 10 per cent of cases (when you see it, it is easily visible under the microscope – it moves around paddled by oar-like flagellae). In the 1970s, we performed a little study at St Thomas' Hospital to examine men whose partners had TV, not just by taking the normal urethral sample but, in addition, massaging the prostate gland through the rectum and massaging the urethra after a metal rod had been passed down the shaft of the penis (the patients had all given their permission). With these extra tests we were able to boost the percentage of positives from 10 per cent to 35 per cent, demonstrating that the TV *was* present in more cases than we were routinely finding. However this investigatory regime would be unacceptable as normal practice and it is now customary in all clinics to offer treatment to men whose partners have TV without having to find the protozoon first.

*Candida albicans*, the cause of thrush, can sometimes give signs that suggest NSU. When this fungus causes a balanitis (inflammation of the foreskin), posthitis (inflammation of the glans penis), or balano-posthitis (inflammation of both), there is often an associated urethritis. This sort of NSU will resolve when the inflammation on the outside of the penis gets better; and is not sensibly treated with antibiotics. However, it is, as ever, not as simple as that, and men may find that they are given antibiotics at the same time as their antifungal cream when thrush is the only condition present. Why do doctors prescribe antibiotics in such circumstances? Because people can have thrush and chlamydia at the same time and it is considered better (see below) to treat when there is any possibility of chlamydia.

Herpes simplex virus (HSV) is an infrequent cause of recurrent non-specific urethritis if the herpetic ulcers are found in the urethra rather than, as is more usual, on the glans or shaft. As it is not routine to test those with possible NSU for HSV, this is a difficult diagnosis at which to arrive. It is further complicated because herpetic urethritis appears to get better with antibiotic treatment. As the natural history of herpes infections is to heal within a week or ten days, this improvement will coincide with the average length of NSU treatment. Once this has happened on a few occasions, the patient will be quite convinced that it is the antibiotics rather than nature that have effected the cure.

## Foreign bodies

It seems to be a human characteristic that men and women, boys and girls, little babies even, take pleasure in inserting odd bits and pieces into available holes and orifices. This pastime, innocent enough in childhood (although keeping the emergency room staff busy), takes on a different significance in adulthood in a sexual context. The inserted objects are known as foreign bodies, a reference to their extra-corporeal rather than their overseas provenance. The vagina is a popular orifice – dildoes are harmless foreign bodies – but the urethra and rectum are sites that can be fraught with problems when used in this way for sexual gratification. Several years ago, a learned surgical journal carried a serious piece about a number of patients with 'vibrating umbilicus syndrome' which emanated from the lower bowel. This self-limiting condition (the batteries ran down) resulted from it being easier to insert a vibrator than to get it out.

### Case history

Freddie P, a 53-year-old, single accountant turned up in the accident and emergency department of a local hospital complaining that, for the past four days, he had noticed beads of pus at the tip of his penis when he woke up in the morning. He had also noticed a burning sensation at the tip of his penis every time he passed urine. When Freddie was examined there was a visible urethral discharge and also a hard tender swelling at the base of the penis and we raised the possibility of a foreign body. Mr P strongly denied inserting anything into his penis and he was sent off for an X-ray of the offending organ. This showed a radio-opaque object which was at first difficult to identify. When shown the X-ray, however, Freddie came clean and explained all. It seemed that he used to insert a safety-pin into his urethra 'for the purposes of masturbation' and attached a length of cotton to it so that he could more easily retrieve it. One day the inevitable happened and the cotton broke. Instead of allowing nature to take its course – it would probably have passed quite easily the next time he peed – he had panicked and tried to manipulate the safety-pin out. Not surprisingly, the pin had sprung open under this onslaught and landed Mr P in a painful and embarrassing situation that required a surgeon's intervention to sort out. Foreign bodies as a cause of urethral discharge in men only make up a very small proportion of cases of NSU seen in clinic.

## What are the symptoms of NSU in men?

The second major problem associated with NSU is, paradoxically, its paucity of symptoms and their minor nature. The symptoms are often so slight that they overlap those that a completely healthy man may have in the absence of any infection at all. This means that a man with an infection may dismiss the symptoms because they are so slight. Conversely, and this is more common, a healthy man, who has had a genuine infection in the past, may constantly think that the infection has returned and go to his clinic (or clinics) in search of further antibiotic cure. He may be successful in procuring repeated courses of treatment because of the lack of precision in diagnosing NSU (see above). After a series of such visits, each accompanied by: 'Just take these tablets; no sex or alcohol, and make sure your girl-friend/wife attends for treatment', it is not surprising that some men start examining themselves minutely every morning and take the slightest tingle when they pee as a sign of infection. The NSU neurosis has set in.

Any small textbook or teaching aid will tell you that NSU and gonorrhoea share the same two main symptoms: dysuria (pain, stinging, burning, discomfort on passing urine) and urethral discharge, the passing of fluid from the urethra. There is, however, a marked difference between the two diagnoses in the severity of these symptoms. Neither gonorrhoea nor NSU gives very severe dysuria these days but there is less likely to be discomfort of any sort with NSU. Likewise, the discharge with NSU is usually scanty, often only present first thing in the morning, compared with the often profuse, purulent discharge associated with gonorrhoea.

It is rare for the discharge of NSU to stain or mark the underwear and it may only become apparent if the urethra is massaged or 'milked' (sometimes by the patient himself when attempting to demonstrate an infection).

No, the symptoms of NSU are mild, often not qualitatively different from normality. If there is no measurable or visible discharge, and the dysuria consists of the slightest 'tingle' when peeing, there is a good chance that there is no significant infection. The trouble is that this lack of discharge and minimal dysuria may be all that is found with chlamydial urethritis, which is what that mild NSU may turn out to be when the chlamydia test comes back from the laboratory.

In spite of great efforts over the years, nobody has been able to differentiate the range of symptoms associated with chlamydia-negative NSU from those associated with proven chlamydial urethritis.

## Non-specific genital infection in women

So, we have a group of conditions which cause NSU/NGU in men, some of which *are* definitely infectious, like chlamydia and TV; some of which *may* be infectious, like *M. genitalium*; some of which are *not* infectious, like alcohol; and some of which are incidental, like thrush. The trouble is that, when the man bowls up to the clinic, we cannot tell which is which. It has been generally accepted that, if a man is diagnosed with NSU, he should organize that his partner is also treated (a) soon and (b) certainly before they have sex again, in case there *is* an infection and he catches it back again. However, she may not be too pleased to be asked to attend the clinic, particularly if she feels fine.

## What are the symptoms of NSGI in women?

Women with uncomplicated non-specific infection are likely to experience no symptoms at all. Indeed, most diagnoses of NSGI are made in asymptomatic women irrespective of whether chlamydia is identified at a later date or not. It seems that chlamydial infection is sometimes associated with an increase or alteration in vaginal discharge but there do not seem to be any particular characteristics of the discharge to help identify chlamydia as a cause.

When a woman with chlamydial infection is examined internally, one can sometimes see changes on the cervix. A muco-purulent discharge may be seen coming from the os, the little hole that marks the entrance to the uterus, and there may or may not be an area of redness. Although when one sees the discharge from the os (likened sometimes to a waterfall) there is immediate suspicion of the possibility of chlamydial infection, it is probably true that in most cases there is no characteristic 'look' to the cervix.

If chlamydia is present in the cervix, the inflammation that it causes can result in some inter-menstrual bleeding (IMB) which may be noticed following sexual intercourse. There are other reasons that women may bleed between their periods but, if spotting or bleeding does occur, it is certainly worth excluding chlamydial infection. But remember, most women with chlamydia do not notice any bleeding and most cases of bleeding are not due to chlamydial infection.

Because, more often than not, chlamydia presents a lack of clues from itself, women may sometimes believe that symptoms due to another condition are actually due to chlamydia. For example, 'I know I've got chlamydia because of the smell' or 'as soon as the itching came, I knew he'd been up to his old tricks again and given me chlamydia'. In the first case BV had previously occurred at the same time as chlamydia; in the second it had been thrush.

It is this lack of symptoms, at least until complications have set in (by which time damage may have been done), that makes chlamydial infection such a worry for women. Getting a chlamydia test done at the GP, Family Planning or GUM clinic, whenever there has been a possibility or likelihood of infection is sensible advice, always remembering that the more tests that are done, the greater the chance of a result being falsely positive.

## How do we manage non-specific infection?

Specialists working in clinics fully recognize that many of the people who are treated for non-specific infections probably don't need the treatment – men because their NSU is not the infectious sort and, likewise, women because their partner's NSU is not infectious. Our difficulty is in deciding into which category the men and women fall. Although men in general are less likely to suffer significantly if their NSU is not treated, women run the risk of serious complications if a genuine infection is not treated, as the next chapter on complications explains. As a rule, we would rather over-treat than under-treat.

We prefer to examine a woman whose partner has NSU rather than just giving the treatment as it is possible that we may find something that gives us a clue as to the exact diagnosis. TV and candida are two such diagnoses as neither is found as readily in men as in women and, particularly when a man is suffering from repeated, recurrent, attacks of NSU, finding either of these in the female partner can save much time and angst.

The diagnosis of NSU using pus cell counts has been referred to earlier in the chapter and there persists a real dilemma in terms of management. Taking *Chlamydia trachomatis*, we are left with an undoubted pathogen which causes a urethritis with the production of pus cells in the majority of cases. But not all. So we are left with the bizarre situation in which somebody with undoubted inflammation in the urethra may have no infection, while somebody with no signs of urethritis may be infected. No wonder many patients who have had NSU become confused and even neurotic about their condition.

## Case history

James B, a 35-year-old single graphic designer, had never thought of himself as promiscuous and preferred his consecutive monogamous relationships to the idea of a succession of one night stands. He had had more than 30 different partners during his 18 years of sexual activity and had always used condoms but usually only at the start of a new relationship. He was aware of STIs and knew that condoms prevented their spread but as he had never had any symptoms, he had never seen the need to have himself screened for infection. He reckoned VD was something that happened to other people and was somewhat surprised when he developed a scanty urethral discharge seven weeks after sleeping with his new girlfriend, Liz, who was younger than him and relatively sexually inexperienced. They had used condoms for the first three weeks of the relationship. His last sexual experience before meeting Liz had been four months previously and she had not slept with anyone else during the nine months since she had broken up with her previous boyfriend with whom she had been going out for a year.

One week before he attended the clinic, James had noticed a little discoloured stain on his underpants before going to bed and a little clear mucous at the tip of his penis first thing the following morning. Now that his brain was concentrating on his genitalia, he was aware of a slight burning sensation when he passed water. It was a week before he could find the time to attend the local clinic where microscopy of a urethral smear confirmed the diagnosis of NSU and he was prescribed seven days of tetracycline (doxycycline) and advised to abstain from sex. Liz was seen the following day and although nothing was found at her initial examination, she was also treated, this time with four capsules taken just once (azithromycin). As they had both had other tests (for syphilis, gonorrhoea and HIV infection), they returned together two weeks later to pick up their results. All their tests, including chlamydia, turned out to be negative. James' slight discharge had got better and Liz had noticed that her vaginal discharge, which she had not thought in any way abnormal, had lessened.

All was well for the next fortnight until James telephoned the clinic to say that his infection had returned. At his insistence he was seen the same day and a full examination failed to reveal any abnormality. He was still convinced that there was something wrong and said that he had noticed some discharge in the morning and a slight 'tingle' when he first passed urine in the day. He had got into the habit of examining himself minutely every day and would squeeze and 'milk' his urethra to see if there was any sign of discharge. When he found that he could demonstrate some discharge in the early mornings he was convinced that his infection had returned, not realizing that the majority of males can produce a little bit of mucus at the urethral meatus in the morning, if they try.

In this case a budding urethral neurosis was nipped before it could really blossom. Often, however, an attack of non-specific urethritis can be followed by months, if not years, of needless worry and anxiety simply because, following the mind's focusing on the genitalia, the patient has noticed certain characteristics of his sexual organs for the first time, and normality has become abnormality.

## Treatment of NSGI

The drugs used in the treatment of non-specific infection have varied little over the years although the length of time that they are taken has changed. The very first antimicrobial agents, sulphonamides, were thought to be effective from their inception and were still in use in the 1970s when I first began to treat NSU and when *Chlamydia trachomatis* had only just been discovered. In those days tetracyclines were the first line of treatment and were often given for three weeks. The other alternative was erythromycin, a macrolide antibiotic, also given for two to three weeks. It was further proof of chlamydia's role in NSU when it was found in the laboratory to be killed by tetracycline and erythromycin.

Over the years the length of treatment has changed, usually downwards, and, at the time of writing, most clinics now use a tetracycline (doxycycline) twice a day for one week or a newish macrolide, azithromycin, which has the considerable advantage of being taken all in one go on the day the diagnosis is made. Abstinence from sex is important during treatment to stop re-infection or further transmission before the antibiotics have had time to work.

Some tetracyclines, particularly the more modern ones such as doxycycline, can make the skin particularly sensitive to sunlight (or sun beds) and are also prone to giving a painful oesophagitis if not fully swallowed. Hence the advice on taking treatment comprises three 'S's: no sex, swallow carefully with food and avoid bright sunlight (or use a strong sun block).

The no-alcohol rule was steadfastly applied back in the 1970s without any convincing medical rationale. Whether or not this reflected an old-fashioned 'punitive' approach to medicine, men up and down the country, known for their ten-pint capacity or love for fine wine were receiving old-fashioned looks as they asked for a half-pint of lime juice or a 'tonic on its own, please'.

Some experts in NSU (patients, that is) voluntarily cut down their alcohol intake because of its potential inflammatory effects on the urethra but there have been no scientific trials showing that consumption of alcohol delays the resolution of NSU.

## Resources

www.bashh.org/guidelines.htm

# 6 Non-specific genital infection: complications

The complications of non-specific infection took up all of a page and a half in the 1979 edition of this book and there wasn't even an entry for pelvic inflammatory disease in the index. The topic was covered in relation to gonococcal infection, along with ectopic pregnancy and pelvic pain, but the overwhelming contribution of *Chlamydia trachomatis* was not then as clear to either the medical profession or the general public as it is today. So, at the start of the third millennium, complications warrant a chapter to themselves.

## What are the complications of non-specific genital infection?

The complications focus around those associated with chlamydial infection. The genus *Chlamydia* is made up of various species of which three are pathogenic to humans. *Chlamydia trachomatis* is divided into fifteen different types named after letters of the alphabet. D to K are those (technically called the 'oculo-genital' sort) that cause non-specific urethritis. Types A, B and C cause trachoma, an infectious eye condition which affects close on 500 million people worldwide. The various 'L' types of *Chlamydia* cause lymphogranuloma venereum (LGV) which is dealt with in Chapter 10. *Chlamydia psittaci* is primarily a bird pathogen but can infect humans giving psittacosis ('parrot-fancier's lung'). *Chlamydia pneumoniae* is the final human pathogen, causing lung infections. It has also been associated with atherosclerosis and heart disease.

### Eye disease

We see then that the chlamydia that causes NSU is closely related to one of the leading world causes of blindness, trachoma, so it is no surprise that the sexually transmitted form can infect the eye as well as the genitalia.

Conjunctivitis is a relatively infrequent complication and follows contamination of the eye by genital secretions. There may be quite a lot of purulent discharge from underneath the eyelids which, themselves, can be seen to be red and inflamed when pulled back. The eye infection in turn can spread to the middle ear (otitis media) with a temporary hearing loss. This is uncommon. Unlike other inflammatory or infective eye conditions, chlamydial inclusion conjunctivitis (to give it its full name) needs to be treated with oral antibiotics in addition to any local ointments or creams. It will resolve without any lasting damage unless left untreated for several months. If an eye condition is diagnosed as chlamydial, it is obviously crucial to investigate and treat any sexual partners, however unlikely the link between the eye and the nether regions may seem.

## Reactive arthritis

What used to be called Reiter's disease, or sometimes Reiter's syndrome, comprises a triad of conditions: arthritis, conjunctivitis and urethritis (NSU), and had been recognized two centuries before Hans Reiter described it in troops in trenches in the First World War. Reiter's disease seemed to be provoked by either sexual intercourse or dysentery and even in the post-dysenteric form there was a marked urethritis, giving the abstinent monk with food-poisoning some explaining to do.

There are five bacteria accepted as causing a reactive arthritis: *Salmonella* (typhoid), *Shigella, Campylobacter* and *Yersinia* (dysentery and diarrhoea), and *Chlamydia trachomatis*. In our practice we mostly see patients whose symptoms have followed sex and their condition is a subdivision of reactive arthritis with the sweetly named acronym SARA (for sexually acquired reactive arthritis). Possibly up to a half of SARA cases are 'provoked' by chlamydial infection as evidenced by identification of the organism itself, or bits of it, in joint fluid. Most people with a chlamydia-induced arthritis go first to the rheumatologist, eye doctor or skin specialist and will have had their original infection eliminated by the time they see the GUM physician.

The urethritis and arthritis can be accompanied by eye problems (conjunctivitis or uveitis) and skin problems (keratodermia blennorhagica, a thickening of the skin on the feet, and circinate balanitis, shiny red blotches on the glans penis).

SARA has a couple of confusing aspects. Firstly, given that the condition is likely to have followed chlamydial infection, the conjunctivitis is, surprisingly, not directly caused by chlamydia. Secondly, while it is obviously important to treat the initial provoking chlamydial urethritis with antibiotics, further flare-ups of the urethritis are not infective and do not need any further such treatment. This is because all the manifestations of the condition, the arthritis, eye problems, urethritis, etc., are part of an auto-immune reaction to the original infection. In this, the immune system mistakes bits of healthy body for the bacterium. Although it takes a bacterial infection to set the process off, once started no reinfection is needed to keep it going. Imagine a ball travelling down an incline. Once the ball has started to move, gravity takes over and while it might slow down or speed up depending on the slope, no further pushing is required.

Not everybody who gets chlamydial infection develops SARA. Of those who *do* develop reactive arthritis, 60–80 per cent carry a tissue antigen called HLA B27, compared with less than 10 per cent in the general population. *Chlamydia trachomatis* is the trigger but, as with any gun, it only needs to be pulled once for the bullet to be on its way.

## Chlamydial infection in babies

Ophthalmia neonatorum is the Latin name for the 'sticky eye' that is seen in newborn babies soon after birth and, in the old days, was most often due to gonorrhoea acquired from the mother during delivery. Today in the UK the gonococcal variety is outnumbered 5 to 1 by chlamydial ophthalmia. Whereas eye infection in the newborn caused by gonorrhoea comes on a day or two after birth, when mother and child are still in hospital, chlamydial conjunctivitis may take a week or longer to appear, by which time both are probably back at home.

As with adult eye infection, systemic (oral) antibiotic treatment is required because, like adults, the infection may spread to the ears and also because it may spread to the lungs. This neonatal chlamydial pneumonitis shows itself a little later, perhaps four or five weeks after delivery and would normally be prevented by the earlier treatment of the eye infection. However, perhaps half the babies with chlamydial lung infection have had no symptoms of eye or ear trouble before they develop their cough and rapid breathing. It is important to make the diagnosis as early as possible as babies who have suffered from chlamydial pneumonitis are more likely to have problems with bronchitis and asthma later in life.

Just as the number of cases of gonococcal ophthalmia neonatorum can serve as an indirect measure of how well that disease is being controlled in a community (see Chapter 4) so the incidence of neonatal chlamydial infection gives an indication of the success or otherwise of national chlamydia screening campaigns.

# Complications in women

The medical complications of chlamydial infection in women are both more frequent and more serious than those in men and, not surprisingly, they revolve around aspects of reproductive health. In uncomplicated chlamydial infection the bacterium is found in and around the cervix uteri, the neck of the womb (usually referred to simply as the cervix). Confined to the cervix, chlamydia does no harm although it obviously has the potential to infect any male organ which happens to be in the vicinity. Problems arise when the infection spreads further internally to involve the uterus itself, the fallopian tubes and other pelvic contents.

## Pelvic inflammatory disease (PID or pelvic infection)

As a result of a plethora of gruesome leaflets and handouts and other efforts of health educators, pelvic infection with its sequelae of ectopic pregnancy, infertility and life-long pelvic pain, is the diagnosis most feared by women attending the GUM clinic. Genuine pelvic infection undoubtedly occurs much less frequently than would appear from the number of diagnoses reported from these specialist units for reasons given in the previous chapter. In brief, we would rather overtreat than miss cases. However, a mistake is often made by the clinician when talking to the patient about their diagnosis. I make a point, as I hand out the advice and antibiotics, of saying 'I am treating you for a *possible* pelvic infection'. We cannot be sure about the diagnosis at this stage and, in many cases, may never be certain (see below), but it is important to voice this doubt rather than attach a label that is perceived by the patient as a life sentence with hard labour.

The label PID encompasses a spectrum of conditions assumed to be caused, initially at any rate, by infection. Infection can spread up from the cervix to involve the endometrium, the lining of the uterus, and then spread along the fallopian tubes which connect the uterus to the pelvic cavity where the ovaries lie. The fallopian tubes, one on each side for each ovary, provide a channel for the ovum to travel on its way to the uterus. When successful conception occurs, the egg is fertilized on its way down the tube and will already have divided several times by the time it implants itself in the endometrium. The movement of the egg is helped firstly by peristalsis, a rippling movement not unlike squeezing sausage meat from a sausage, and, secondly, by the action of ciliated cells in the lining of the fallopian tube. Cilia are like little hairs which waft the egg in the right direction.

Although 'blocked' tubes is the diagnosis often given as a cause for infertility, it is more usually damage to the tube rather than actual blockage that is responsible. Destruction of the ciliated lining and fibrosis of the tube following infection, mean that the egg does not travel at the correct speed towards the womb and either arrives at the wrong stage of development and fails to implant, or implants in the wrong place, as with an ectopic pregnancy.

Salpingitis (an '-itis' of the salpynx, the tube) can be acute or chronic. Acute salpingitis is an active and serious infection characterized by fever and severe lower abdominal pain. Chlamydial infection is the most common single cause. Chronic salpingitis gives a more constant pain, without fever, and may or may not be associated with active infection, although it is usual to give antibiotics to be safe. The pain of salpingitis, acute or chronic, is exacerbated by sexual intercourse, so-called 'deep dyspareunia'.

Infection can spread on through the fallopian tubes and leak out into the pelvic cavity itself, where it can involve the ovaries and cause a build-up of pus or fluid in the area. Once this has happened, even after all traces of infection have been eliminated by antibiotics, there often remains 'sticky' inflammation from the fluid. This can cause bits and pieces of tissue in the pelvis to be stuck together by 'adhesions', rather like a fly tied up in a spider's web. These adhesions often develop gradually over months or even years and are themselves a cause of chronic pelvic pain and deep dyspareunia.

## Case history

Kylie M was a 15-year-old schoolgirl who had been in a steady sexual relationship with her 19-year-old boyfriend for three years. Although such a sexual liaison is illegal in the UK, it was condoned by Kylie's mother who regarded Wayne as the son she had never had and allowed him to sleep over three or four times a week. One Friday, when Kylie had endured eight hours of increasing lower abdominal pain, she, her mother and her boyfriend attended the local accident and emergency (A&E) department where, after a four-hour wait, she was seen, examined and sent home with paracetamol and advice to rest. When asked, she had told the doctor that her recent periods had been normal and on time. She returned to the hospital on Saturday evening rather worse, was examined and again sent home with painkillers. At her visit on Sunday afternoon, she was examined yet again, a sexual history was taken for the third time and a diagnosis of possible pelvic infection was made. She was advised to come back on Monday morning to attend the GUM department where she could have a full examination for STIs and get the appropriate treatment.

Although it was 'appointments only' that morning, it was obvious when Kylie and her mother turned up that Kylie was very unwell – she could barely walk and was doubled up with pain, and she was seen almost immediately. When she was examined her abdomen was rigid and she cried when it was simply touched by a gentle hand. If you put your ear to a healthy person's stomach, you will hear gurgling noises ('borborygmi' for the technically minded) which are evidence that the intestines are working correctly (doctors use a stethoscope). There was no noise at all coming from Kylie's abdomen. There was a stale smell on her breath (fetor), she had been sick and had not had a bowel movement since Friday.

Kylie was in the surgical operating theatre within two hours where her burst appendix was removed and the inside of her abdominal cavity, the site of her peritonitis, cleaned and mopped out.

Kylie's age and her admitted sexual relationship with a young adult had blinded the staff in A&E to diagnosis which would have been easy for a first-year medical student – acute appendicitis.

## Infertility

The risks of infertility increase with each infection involving the fallopian tubes and when there is delay in starting treatment for proven chlamydia. Older women seem to suffer more problems than younger but it is the number of episodes that has the greatest effect on subsequent ability to conceive. One estimate suggests that 10 per cent are infertile after one attack, 20 per cent after two and 40 per cent after three diagnoses of tubal PID.

These figures are probably unduly pessimistic as they refer to proven episodes of acute salpingitis, a diagnosis, as detailed below, that is comparatively rare.

## What are the causes of PID?

We have seen that *Chlamydia trachomatis* is an important culprit with the gonococcus also implicated, more so in some countries than others. However, between them, these two organisms are found in less than half the cases analysed in the UK, perhaps 40 per cent at maximum. In other countries with higher levels of infection, gonorrhoea has been found in up to 80 per cent and chlamydial infection in up to 50 per cent of cases. A well-conducted prospective study, published in the USA in 1996, demonstrated convincingly that screening (and treating) young women for chlamydia drastically reduced the incidence of pelvic infection.

Some authorities have suggested the germs found in bacterial vaginosis (Chapter 3) are responsible for a number of cases. The evidence is unconvincing although metronidazole (the normal treatment for BV on its own) is commonly prescribed in addition to other antibiotics in cases of PID.

There is quite good evidence that *Mycoplasma hominis*, the short-lived cause of NSU (see previous chapter), is responsible for some cases, and those who support *Mycoplasma genitalium*'s role in NSU believe it may also be responsible for some cases of pelvic infection.

## What are symptoms and signs of PID?

Here we run into real difficulty. A clinical diagnosis (the diagnosis made at a visit to the doctor) is made by assessing the *symptoms*, what the patient has noticed, and the *signs*, what the doctor finds on examining the patient. In Chapter 2, when discussing laboratory tests, we looked at the concepts of *sensitivity*, how efficiently will the test pick up positives, and *specificity*, how likely is the positive result to be true? In pelvic inflammatory disease, taking the symptoms and signs to be tests (has the patient got PID, and is it actually PID?), we find the sensitivity and the specificity of both are very low.

This means that, if a patient has PID, they may have *no* signs or symptoms. This is bad news because the infection can go on damaging the pelvic organs while giving no warning or clue to the hapless woman. One expert has suggested that two-thirds of cases of PID are missed because the signs and symptoms are either absent or very slight.

Alternatively, a woman may attend her physician with 'classic' symptoms and/or signs of pelvic infection yet be suffering from something completely different. It is this difficulty in being certain about the diagnosis that encourages doctors to offer antibiotics if there is the slightest chance that there may be infection in the pelvis.

The textbooks say that vaginal discharge or bleeding, stinging or burning on urination and fever are all symptoms of PID but, at laparoscopy (looking inside the abdominal cavity with a tiny telescope), women with these symptoms are found to have normal fallopian tubes as often as infected ones. The same lack of difference is found with blood tests including white cell count and other measures of infection.

Pelvic, lower abdominal pain, remains the mainstay of diagnosis and is the symptom that most often brings the patient to the clinic. There may also be an unusual, for that woman, amount of period pain, dysmenorrhoea. It appears that during the menstrual period, infection is more likely to ascend (move up from the cervix to uterus and then tubes). In many women it has been noticed incidentally that there is a retrograde, backwards, flow of menstrual blood during the period. Indeed, this is thought to be the cause of some cases of dysmenorrhoea as blood irritates the peritoneum. This backwards flow could easily carry infectious bugs, gonorrhoea or chlamydia, with it. Whatever the explanation, the pain of gonococcal pelvic infection has been shown to come on in many cases at the end of, or immediately following, a period.

Indirect evidence for the difficulty in diagnosis is seen when one compares the number of appendectomies performed in boys and girls, young men and women, at different ages. It remains the same for both sexes throughout childhood until soon after puberty. Then the girls streak ahead with twice as many operations on the appendix. This disparity continues until the mid-twenties when men and women converge to have approximately the same rates of diagnosis. Why are females in the 15–25-years age range more likely to have appendicitis? Well, of course, they are not more likely. The extra operations coincide directly with the period when teenagers and young women are most likely to catch chlamydia, develop pelvic infection with belly ache and be misdiagnosed as cases of appendicitis.

So, what is one to do? Women who worry that they may have PID should consult their doctor or go to a clinic, and, as previously mentioned, they might be treated as a *possible* case of PID. A case of 'better safe than sorry'. It is the practice in GUM clinics to see and examine (and usually treat) the sexual partners of women with possible PID and this cycle of events should not be taken, by either partner, as evidence of a sexually transmitted infection with all its implications for the relationship.

Finally, a rare complication of pelvic infection is spread to tissue surrounding the liver, a perihepatitis, known as Fitzhugh-Curtis syndrome. This was originally described following gonorrhoea but today is more likely to be associated with chlamydial infection. It used to be thought that there was direct spread from the pelvis to the liver via an anatomical channel called the right paracolic gutter. Fine in women, but men don't have one, yet do occasionally suffer from Fitzhugh-Curtis syndrome. Spread along lymphatic channels is probably the route but, whatever is correct, it is a diagnosis that is missed more often than not. This is because pain in the top right-hand side of the abdomen, over the liver, would not make doctors or patients think of a sexually transmitted disease, and the usual, mistaken, diagnosis is of cholecystitis.

## What other conditions cause pelvic pain?

Probably the most common reason for lower abdominal pain in young women is endometriosis. As its name implies, this condition relates to the lining of the uterus, the endometrium, which is the tissue into which the fertilized ovum implants itself after conception. The blood-rich endometrium starts to grow after each menstrual period but, if no egg has implanted, sheds itself, usually once a month, giving the 'period'.

For reasons nobody understands, bits of endometrium, instead of being shed and washed away at the end of each cycle, attach themselves to other bits of tissue in the pelvis, perhaps during the retrograde flow mentioned earlier. These bits of endometrium can be found on the ovaries or adjoining segments of lower bowel and stick there after the period has finished. Sometimes pieces of endometrium are found further away from the pelvis and may have reached these sites by blood spread or along lymphatics. They are under the same hormonal influence as the proper endometrium inside the uterus, and so will enlarge, engorge and then shed in the same way, as the cycle progresses, except that they are in the wrong anatomical position. Quite excruciating lower abdominal pain ensues usually, but not always, related to the timing of the period.

Ovarian cysts, little balloons of fluid on the surface of the ovary, are common and can cause sharp pains when they rupture.

Ectopic pregnancy is one cause of pain that it is important not to miss. We have seen how, following damage to the fallopian tubes, the fertilized ovum may not be delivered on time to its natural site of implantation because of damage or blockage in the tubes. If it implants elsewhere, it stimulates whatever tissue it is on to provide blood vessels, rather in the way the placenta grows in a normal gestation.

What works well inside the uterus is a literally life-threatening disaster if bowel or fallopian tubes are involved. As the ectopic pregnancy progresses, the blood supply becomes more than the delicate fallopian or bowel tissue can support and massive bleeding occurs. As this starts, there is significant lower abdominal pain and, unless dealt with as an emergency, there is a real risk of bleeding to death. When an ectopic pregnancy occurs in a tube, it usually has to be removed in the life-saving operation, a unilateral salpingectomy. Surprisingly, however, many women go on to conceive and bear children even though they only have one tube left.

Many of those who have previously had pelvic infection get recurrent bouts of lower abdominal pain over the years. It may be assumed that they have caught yet another infection and some end up being treated with antibiotics on a regular basis, year after year. The suggestion that they are catching yet more STIs, apart from being soul-destroying, does nothing for what is probably a completely faithful relationship. Even the repeatedly negative tests for chlamydia and gonorrhoea do little to reassure women caught in this situation. The adhesions referred to earlier are a likely cause in these circumstances and it may take a laparoscopy to confirm the diagnosis.

## What of the future?

You will have gathered that today's diagnosis and management of possible pelvic inflammatory disease is unsatisfactory. Researchers have recently re-examined how well the clinical diagnosis correlates with the diagnosis at laparoscopy and found it to be even worse than first thought. Further, even laparoscopy has lost some of its conviction as it is now realized that there may be significant infection inside a fallopian tube that appears quite normal – in one series, 12 of 27 women with ectopic pregnancy had quite normal-looking tubes.

On the positive side, there have been advances in X-ray departments, using sophisticated modern scanners and some of the newer blood tests, for example, looking at special antibodies to chlamydial heat-shock proteins, seem to offer more specific results than the old-fashioned ones.

## Treatment of PID

In the UK it is rare to see acute 'hot' cases of salpingitis in GUM departments, these tending to go to A&E and on to gynaecologists. Once a provisional diagnosis has been made (this will be before the STI test results are available), antibiotic treatment should be started as early as possible and usually lasts for at least two weeks. Tetracyclines or macrolides, like erythromycin, are the first line of treatment and metronidazole is often added. Other antibiotics include cephalosporins and quinolones. Whichever drugs are used, rest is recommended, preferably in bed, preferably alone.

# Complications in men

## Epididymo-orchitis

The epididymis is a tissue attached to the back of the testis which serves as the collecting tube for spermatozoa. At the top of the testis it becomes the spermatic cord which then runs a course to the seminal vesicles, where the sperm are stored. Infection can spread backwards from the urethra along the spermatic cord until it reaches the epididymis and testis. Infection or inflammation of the testicle is called orchitis. When examining a man with a painful swelling in the scrotum, it is difficult to tell whether the process is confined to epididymis on its own or whether the testis is also involved. So, although epididymitis undoubtedly exists on its own, most clinicians prefer to talk of epididymo-orchitis.

In men below the age of forty, the most common infecting organism is *Chlamydia trachomatis*, with the gonococcus a comparative rarity. Over that age, the germs responsible tend to be those associated with UTIs, like *Escherichia coli* or other intestinal bacteria. At the time that a man attends with the signs and symptoms of epididymo-orchitis, there is no way of knowing the causative organism, as is so often the case with PID in women. For that reason, again as with PID, the man's sexual partner is asked to attend and will be examined and probably treated themselves just in case there is chlamydial infection.

Epididymo-orchitis starts with a dull ache in one testicle which progresses over a matter of a few days to much greater discomfort, frank pain and swelling. When the patient is examined in clinic, there is sometimes an associated NSU which may be obvious, with discharge, but more often is only detected on urethral microscopy, if at all. Laboratory tests, including a mid-stream urine (MSU) to see if there is a UTI, are sent off and antibiotics, for two weeks in the first instance, are started. The same antichlamydial agents, tetracyclines and macrolides, are used as for NSU. A suspensory bandage or jock-strap can be worn to ease pressure and relieve pain. For years in my clinic the only sizes available were large, extra large and extra extra large. This at least brought some consolation to the luckless individuals with this painful and worrying condition.

I always warn my patients with this condition that it is likely to go on for at least four weeks. It is important that this should be understood at the beginning because, at the first review after a fortnight of antibiotics, they would otherwise expect a dramatic improvement to have taken place, rather than being prescribed yet another two weeks' worth. In most cases the pain will have resolved and the swelling diminished at four weeks but in some it may take even longer to resolve.

There is some evidence that a bad attack of epididymo-orchitis will affect testicular function and the testicle on the affected side does occasionally end up smaller and softer than before the attack. However, one testicle, like one kidney, is quite enough for normal function and fertility and hormone levels are unaffected.

## What else might it be?

Other swellings of the testicle, with the important exception of torsion, tend not to be tender. A varicocele, which is a collection of redundant blood vessels like varicose veins, usually occurs between the ages of 15 and 26 and is not of clinical significance. It is seen more often on the left side. A hydrocele is a cyst filled with fluid attached to the testis or cord which may increase in size quite dramatically ('the man with three balls') for no apparent reason. Either of these two conditions may produce an ache but not the acute pain of epididymo-orchitis or torsion.

Torsion of the testis is a surgical emergency. Torsion means twisting and this is literally what happens. The testis twists inward from a half-turn to four or five turns which immediately blocks the return of blood in the veins. The testis and epididymis become engorged with blood and gangrene sets in rapidly. If torsion is not operated upon within six to eight hours, the testis will be lost.

The typical patient is a teenager who may have suffered an injury during sport followed by an acute pain which can seem to be coming from the lower abdomen. Other cases occur at night time when again there is sudden onset of severe pain. The affected testicle is very tender and usually hangs higher than normal and flatter (the long axis being horizontal rather than vertical). Occasionally there is a history of recurrent, intermittent similar pain indicating episodes of partial torsion which have righted themselves after a few hours. There is a variation of torsion that occurs in small boys and infants which although anatomically distinct is just as much of an emergency.

If diagnosed in time, a surgeon can untwist the torsion, secure the testis to stop it happening again and secure the testis on the other side. If the testis is dead, it is important to remove because, in a small number of cases, antibodies can develop to the dead tissue which may affect the viable testicle and reduce sperm count and fertility.

## Prostatitis

There is no direct evidence that *Chlamydia trachomatis* is involved in prostatitis, infection/inflammation of the prostate gland, in that chlamydia has never been cultured from the prostate. In a small number of cases the nucleic acid amplification tests have been positive on carefully taken prostatic samples but, if chlamydia is implicated, it is in only a small proportion of cases. The organisms most commonly isolated are those found in urinary tract infections.

Acute prostatitis presents with urinary symptoms similar to cystitis, frequency of micturition, urgency (feeling of needing to pee) and dysuria. In addition symptoms directly from the prostate gland include pain in the rectum, perineum (space between the rectum and scrotum) and penis. If bacteria have entered the bloodstream (rare, but it does occur) fever, muscle and joint pains can occur.

The urinary symptoms can suggest an STI which is why patients with prostatitis turn up in GUM clinics. Chronic prostatitis divides into two types: bacterial, in which, as its name implies, causative micro-organisms are found, and abacterial, also known as chronic pelvic pain syndrome. It is relatively rare to find bacteria in chronic prostatitis. Symptoms include pain in the penis, particularly at the tip, and discomfort in the rectum, perineum and scrotum. Chronic prostatitis should only be diagnosed if the symptoms have been present for at least six months. Treatment is with antibiotics and anti-inflammatory drugs.

A brief word about cancer of the prostate (which is not associated with chlamydial infection). This is the most common cancer in men and there is a vigorous debate at present as to the extent to which screening for early stages should take place. There is a blood test for prostate specific antigen (PSA) which is raised in those with prostate cancer. This test is being promoted in the UK which has a poor five-year survival rate compared with other European countries. However, aggressive treatment of those with raised levels of PSA is very unpleasant for the patient and may be unnecessary as only some 20 per cent of prostate cancers are actually doing any harm to the patient. It is said that a majority of men who die from other causes also happen to have evidence of cancer in their prostates but have suffered no ill effects. So, we are really still waiting for a good test for early harmful prostate cancer. There is a real worry that if more screening tests for PSA are done, there will be more men suffering unnecessarily from the aggressive and debilitating treatment.

## Problems with diagnosis of non-specific infections

Chlamydial infection may not be as common as media reports suggest because of the problems associated with today's methods of diagnosis. In Chapter 2 I talked about ascertainment bias, the difficulty of separating real increases in numbers of cases from an apparent increase simply due to more tests being done. I also tried to explain how a test with a small number of false positive results might appear satisfactory in a group of persons with a high prevalence of infection – most of the positives that are found will be true positives; but that in a low prevalence population, where very few people are infected, *most* of the positives will be false positives.

These various mathematical calculations may serve to guide decision-makers as to where and when to use a given diagnostic test, or indeed, whether to use it at all, and one can persuasively argue that it is better to have a test that picks most of the real infections at the cost of wrongly diagnosing a small proportion as positive. However, it matters not a jot to the person wrongly diagnosed whether they are perceived as belonging to a high or low prevalence population. When this (wrong) diagnosis of chlamydia infection is given to them, its sexual transmission explained and the importance of their partner's attendance for testing and treatment emphasized, a heavy and possibly terminal strain may be put on a relationship. This may not be helped when the partner's test for chlamydia comes back negative.

We regularly see bemused patients in clinic whose chlamydia results are at variance with their partner's. It takes time to try to explain this problem of false positives and, with treatment almost always already having been given, a subsequent negative test does not add, or subtract, credibility to or from the original result. The problem with this widespread, indiscriminate testing for chlamydial infection that is being increasingly rolled out in many countries, is that there is no alternative test that can give a definitive result, as there is with gonorrhoea.

It would probably be generally agreed that the advantages of more testing (diminution of problems with fertility, abdominal pain, ectopic pregnancy, etc.) outweigh the problems that false positives bring to relationships. However, if general testing for chlamydial infection is to continue, it is important that the general public is aware of the limitations of the test. If the screening programmes currently being proposed have the desired effect of diminishing the overall prevalence of chlamydia in the population, the relatively small problem of false positives will make up an even greater proportion of total positives.

## Resources

www.bashh.org/guidelines.htm

# 7 Herpes simplex

By the age of twenty-five, at least 80 per cent of people worldwide have got herpes. That is a statement that needs qualifying but puts this much over-hyped disease in perspective. I often quote an article from the 1970s to the effect that one-third of children are already infected with herpes by the age of three. There are no reliable and equivalent up-to-date figures for this age group, but although the percentage may now be a little lower, the message remains important.

Luckily, the old-fashioned view of herpes as the incurable, frightful, end-of-your-sex-life 'love' virus no longer holds sway in the UK, a result of greater public awareness of the real facts about this common infection. The Herpes Viruses Association, an under-funded and worthy voluntary body in the UK, can take much credit for this change in attitude.

## Herpes simplex viruses (HSV)

There are, at the time of writing, eight different human herpes viruses but the two that concern us here are types 1 and 2 and it is to these two types that I refer when I talk of herpes. Classically type 1 was the one found more usually around the mouth and lips (slightly confusingly called labial herpes after the Latin for lip, *labia*), and type 2 which predominated in the genital and anal area. From the time that these two types were distinguishable from each other, it was recognized that type 1 could infect the genitals and type 2 the mouth but such misalignment was rare. Nowadays, however, genital herpes is more often caused by type 1 than type 2 and this is of both clinical and psychological significance.

## How are herpes viruses caught?

The majority of those infected by HSV worldwide are infected by type 1 on the face or mouth. As most of these infections are asymptomatic, it is impossible to pinpoint the exact event or time when herpes was caught but in many cases it will have been in early childhood and acquired innocently from a parent or other relative who themselves had an active yet asymptomatic oral infection. Unlikely as it is to think of Granny infecting her grandchildren, if it wasn't her it would have been another family member, innocently and unwittingly passing on this most common of viruses.

So, herpes gets passed on by someone who doesn't know they are infected. This is as true for mouth herpes as for genital herpes. For some twenty years I lectured on STIs to two hundred or so young qualified doctors who were training in family planning at the Margaret Pyke Centre in London. The Director, Professor John Guillebaud, used to come into the auditorium when I asked, as I was winding up, 'How many of you have got herpes?' The great professor and I both put our hands up along with perhaps twelve, 6 per cent, of the assembled cream of the medical profession. *Even doctors don't know they've got herpes.*

A survey was carried out in the USA some years ago of women who were known to be positive for HSV-2, the genital sort, where they were asked if they had any symptoms of their infection. About one-half said that they were aware of outbreaks occurring from time to time. Of the other half who said they had no awareness of their infection, one-half (i.e. a quarter of the original number), when told of the symptoms of genital herpes, said that they now recognized that they had had symptoms in the past.

We know about the number of people infected with herpes by means of antibody blood tests which can detect whether an infection has ever been caught in the past and whether it is type 1 or 2 or, in some cases, when both sorts have been acquired. By means of these blood tests it is possible to chart how more and more people become infected as they get older and also how different populations have different degrees of infection. Nobody knows why the prevalences should vary so, but the differences are consistent. Women are more likely to be infected than men, gay men more likely than straight, American more than British, African more than European, European more than those from the Indian sub-continent and so on.

By means of such serological (blood test) surveys it has been possible to chart changes in the numbers infected over the years. Such surveys indicate that fewer young people are infected with HSV today than, say, thirty years ago. A result of this is that more persons have never been exposed to the virus by the time they become sexually active and this may mean a greater proportion of the population is at risk of genital herpes as a result of their first contact with HSV occurring in adulthood.

Genital herpes is a sexually transmitted infection and is caught during sexual contact between an infected individual and one who is not infected.

That bald statement, while true, is the basis for a great deal of unhappiness, anger and resentment and the reason for numerous relationships coming to a precipitate end. In many, perhaps a majority of, cases not only has there been no unfaithfulness to account for the new infection, but the perceived 'offender', he or she who passed on the infection, is the one person with whom a sexual relationship can continue with absolutely no risk of further transmission of HSV. Once you've got it, you can't catch it again.

## Case history

Jane D was looking forward to celebrating the fifth anniversary of her and John's first meeting. They shared a flat, a cat and a mortgage and, apart from a period of three months, three years previously, when they had split up and both had one other partner, had remained sexually and emotionally faithful to one another. One morning she woke up feeling itchy on her left labium, thought no more of it until that evening when she found it rather sore when she peed. The following day the area that had felt itchy was now decidedly painful and it was even more uncomfortable when she passed water. By day three the pain was so bad she found it difficult to sit down and rather than walk, she was waddling.

The family doctor was sympathetic, made a tentative diagnosis of genital herpes and suggested she visit her local GUM clinic. Jane was not best pleased to hear that her 'faithful' partner had infected her with herpes and so attended the local clinic all set to take her partner to the cleaners once the diagnosis had been confirmed. The clinic specialist nurse listened carefully to Jane's tale of woe and, having asked one question, said, 'Your boyfriend has not been unfaithful to you!'

The question she'd asked was: 'Do you and your boyfriend have oral sex – does he go down on you?' to which Jane had answered, 'Yes'. The nurse practitioner then explained that what had almost certainly happened was that her partner had been having a symptom-free attack of labial (mouth) herpes, a cold sore, and had infected her quite unwittingly. Further, it was most likely to be HSV-1 which carried a better outlook, in terms of recurrences, than HSV-2.

People do not intentionally infect other people with sexually transmitted diseases. Genital herpes is one of the two STIs (the other being genital warts, see case history in Chapter 8) which can arise out of the blue in a completely faithful relationship. I regularly see patients who still harbour deep resentment for a past partner, imagining that he or she must have been fully aware of their infection and callously and gratuitously passed it on. As far as this common story of mouth-to-genital transmission is concerned, the truth is different.

# What does the infection do?

As we have seen, in most cases the infection causes no symptoms when it is first acquired. This may be because most infections occur for the first time in childhood and, in common with other virus infections like measles or chicken pox, first attacks are not as bad as when they occur in adults. The first ever attack is known as the *primary* attack. If there are symptoms, they are worse than in any subsequent attack. Because there are no protective antibodies, it takes time for the body to mount a defence against herpes. The virus causes inflammation – itching at first, followed by a blister or blisters at the site of entry, be it the mouth the vulva, penis or anus. There may be quite marked swelling around these sore places. There is a general feeling of unwellness with a fever, aches and pains and swollen glands, particularly those near the site of infection. These may be painful.

The blister(s) burst leaving shallow ulcers that are painful to touch. These will heal after a matter of a few days, in most cases between seven and ten. If the primary site is open to the air, as on the mouth or shaft of the penis, the sore will crust over and be more uncomfortable than if on a covered bit of skin such as under the foreskin or inside the vulva where it can remain moist. A primary attack of genital herpes can be a nasty experience, particularly in women. Urine, as it flows over the sores, can cause pain and this was thought to be the reason for some women having difficulty in peeing. We now know that the herpes virus can actually attack the spinal cord at its lower level (technically, a transverse myelitis) interfering with the nerves that control the ability to micturate and defecate (pee and poo). Difficulty with defecation is rarely an important symptom but inability to urinate sometimes necessitates catherization of the bladder.

Confusingly, someone who was unknowingly infected in the past with HSV may suddenly develop symptoms for the very first time, maybe years later. This is called an *initial* attack and resembles a recurrence rather than a primary attack, that is to say, not as bad.

All people who are infected with herpes (remember, that is most of the adults in the world) will have further outbreaks, or recurrences. For those who were symptomatic with their primary attack, the recurrence is usually recognized as such. It will occur on the same part of the body but is not as severe. It may simply show itself as a temporarily itchy area. The frequency of recurrent attacks varies in different individuals. I recently saw a woman who noticed her first recurrence seven years after her primary infection. At the other end of the spectrum, the first recurrence may run on seamlessly from the primary attack. What one can say with confidence is that, in general, recurrent attacks become less frequent and less severe as time goes by.

It is sometimes difficult to be certain that a recurrence of herpes actually is a recurrence. Surprisingly, the condition most frequently confused with herpes in women is thrush. In probably six or seven out of ten women who consult me because of recurrent genital herpes, the symptoms of soreness are actually due to vulval candidal infection. Of course, the others are indeed having outbreaks of herpes but if the symptoms persist for longer than ten days or seem to be there almost constantly, herpes is very unlikely as the correct diagnosis.

## What brings on a recurrent attack?

Nobody knows for certain – it would be difficult to persuade an ethics committee to sanction a prospective trial which measured the outcomes in susceptible folk of different provocative stimuli – but there is enough anecdotal evidence to have provided a consensus of the most common factors associated with outbreaks of labial and genital herpes.

High body temperature (over 103 degrees Fahrenheit in old parlance, 39.5 Celsius in modern) was recognized in the pre-antibiotic era as a provoker of herpes. In those days, before the Second World War, the consultant on his ward round could diagnose those with lobar pneumonia, always associated with a high fever, from the end of the bed just by noting their outbreak of cold sores.

Too much ultraviolet light is well known to skiers and sun lovers in general as a predisposing factor for cold sores. It would take a particularly dedicated naturist to fall victim to this as a cause of genital herpes although, years ago, I did have a patient whose attacks had virtually ceased until she emigrated to Palm Beach where the high ambient temperature allows the inhabitants to get up to all sorts of mischief on their sunny roofs.

Trauma (from the Greek for wound) is another recognized cause. A biff on the mouth might bring on an attack and, although sexual intercourse is not, under normal circumstances, 'traumatic', some people (this is pretty rare) with genital herpes find that they do get recurrences following sex. If these turn out to be real attacks (see above for thrush as an alternative diagnosis) then prophylactic antiviral therapy will do the trick.

Stress. Although, again, there is no hard evidence on this one, enough people with herpes believe that stress is involved with attacks that it is really impossible to ignore it as a provoking factor. That there is a psychological element to herpes is undoubted. Many years ago there was a trial of a brand new anti-herpes agent which was tried out on those with very frequent recurrences. These sugar tablets (for that is in fact what they were) managed to reduce the number of attacks from an average of six per year to less than two. This sort of trial would not be possible today. Firstly, it would never have passed an ethics committee's perusal because the participants were misled about the antiviral ingredient (sugar by mouth has no direct effect on herpes). Secondly, it is very difficult to find a large number of people with herpes who have such frequent attacks. However, it did demonstrate the power and effect of belief on a physical problem.

## How is genital herpes diagnosed?

The first, and most immediate, diagnosis will be a clinical one. An experienced specialist will in most cases be able to make the diagnosis having listened to the story (the 'history') and examined the area in question. For this sort of diagnosis, and for the more sophisticated ones to follow, there does need to be an attack in progress at the time of examination. Coming to the doctor with a typical story, but three months after the attack when there is nothing to see, is unlikely to allow a definite confirmation of herpes to be made.

Other direct methods of diagnosis again rely on an active sore being present at the time of examination. Growing the virus (inoculated on fresh hens' eggs) has rather gone out of fashion as it is a time-consuming and fiddly process. Direct examination of a sample using an electron microscope has the advantage of speed and immediacy but is not readily available in most centres. More modern techniques now commonly used identify specific herpes DNA and may be able to differentiate between HSV-1 and HSV-2. Most of these tests, apart from the clinical diagnosis and the, usually unavailable, electron microscopy, take some days before a result is ready.

Finally there is serology. These blood tests can tell whether anyone has ever been infected by herpes and whether it is type 1 or type 2, or both. However, unless the infection is very recent, when a different and transient sort of antibody is found, the blood test cannot tell how long the infection has been present or, indeed, whether the site of infection is mouth or genitals. Many clinics, including my own, do not offer herpes serology as a routine. There are some cases, for example, when one partner is a known positive and the other's status is unknown, when crucial life and relationship decisions are thought to depend on the outcome of serological testing.

However, there is disagreement as to how useful this test is as a routine and some worries lest the result is used inappropriately to determine the real risks of future transmission. As has been emphasized in earlier chapters when discussing tests for gonorrhoea and chlamydial infection, the prevalence of infection in a given population makes a lot of difference to the usefulness of the test, particularly regarding false positives. In the general population of the UK, up to 40 per cent of positives will be false positives and, even in those attending an STD clinic, that figure will be around 10 per cent. And, of course, there will be a small number of false negatives.

## How likely am I to pass on herpes?

Not very, is the simple answer, particularly if common sense is allowed to prevail. As we have seen, almost everybody has herpes, a majority with infection of the lips or mouth, almost all of which are type 1. If someone who already has HSV-1 is exposed to their sexual partner's herpes virus, as long as that is also type 1, no reinfection can occur. You cannot catch the same virus twice. It is true that there exists a very small minority of people who are infected with both HSV-1 and HSV-2 but they remain just that – a very small minority. Common sense comes into play with regard to when not to have sex. Clearly it would be silly (however small the risk, to say nothing of any possible discomfort) to have sexual contact when you knew you had an outbreak of herpes, labial or genital.

Some people with genital herpes have entered into long and rewarding relationships with others with the same condition, happy in the knowledge that there is no chance of passing herpes on however often they have unprotected sex.

What is true for HSV is not, unfortunately, true for HIV infection, where the other person's virus may be resistant to all sorts of antiviral agents and there is a risk that it takes over from your own less virulent type.

## What is the treatment of genital herpes?

The treatment of a primary attack of genital herpes differs from that of a recurrence because the primary attack is usually much more severe. It has been noted that women are likely to suffer from their symptoms rather more than men – for what are probably simple anatomical reasons. One needs therefore to treat not just the infection itself but also the complications that may have resulted from it.

More than twenty years ago an antiviral treatment was introduced, aciclovir, which literally revolutionized the treatment of herpes simplex infections. Taken five times daily for five days it had a dramatic effect on the symptoms and on the duration of the attack. For the first time there was a magic bullet available for the primary attack and, joy of joys, hope for those who had been crippled by frequent recurrences of their genital herpes. Admittedly, it was rather inconvenient in its dosage regimen, remembering a tablet three times daily is hard enough, let alone five times, but many were more than happy to put up with this minor difficulty.

Aciclovir, or the more modern variations on it, do not in themselves attend to all the problems that can accompany a primary attack of genital herpes. Acute retention of urine, when it is simply not possible to pee at all, is a serious and painful condition necessitating drainage of the bladder in some other way. A tube can be inserted directly into the bladder through a hole in the lower abdominal wall (a supra-pubic catheter), or up through the urethra, to let out the urine. This can lead to introduction of bacteria into the bladder and subsequent cystitis and is therefore to be avoided if possible.

Before the decision is taken to drain the bladder with a catheter, it is often possible to manage by other means. Trying to pee in a warm bath very often does the trick particularly when combined with an application of an anaesthetic ointment or gel, such as lignocaine (lidocaine). This can be quite useful anyway during a primary attack to alleviate what can be quite severe pain.

In the old days, the main limiting factor in the use of aciclovir (acyclovir as it was then) was its cost. Eighty pounds for a five-day course (perhaps £140 or $200 at today's prices) was simply too much for many depart-ments' budgets and its use usually had to be restricted to primary attacks unless the patient could afford to pay for their own medication.

When the patent for aciclovir ran out in the 1990s, almost immediately there came on the market a number of copies of aciclovir (these are tech-nically called 'generic' aciclovir) at greatly reduced price, so making it available for much more widespread use, in particular for suppressive therapy. In addition to the cheap generic aciclovir, other new antivirals were also released, notably valaciclovir and famciclovir. These had the advantage of needing to be taken less frequently than aciclovir but the dis-advantage of being very expensive compared with the, now affordable, generic aciclovir copies.

Suppressive therapy is a treatment designed to stop recurrences of herpes. It is of use in that minority who are troubled by very frequent attacks and has revolutionized the lives of such sufferers. Given in a more convenient dosage (currently 400 mg twice daily) it simply stops recurrences. There appear to be no long-term problems with continuous aciclovir and some people have taken it for many years without side-effects or complications.

Aciclovir is also used successfully in some people as abortive therapy. When used in this way, it is taken the very instant that there is a sign of a fresh attack beginning. For those in whom this works, the tablets literally abort the oncoming attack before it has had a chance to take hold. Tablets are taken for three to four days only. It doesn't suit everybody but, in those who get a reliable warning of an impending attack, it works well and does mean there is no need to take medication continuously as in suppressive therapy.

Unless taken as described (i.e. immediately a recurrence starts) aciclovir or the more modern anti-herpes drugs do not have any significant effect on recurrent attacks and, if taken two or three days into an attack, are unlikely to make any difference either to the severity or length of an attack.

We are often asked if there are medical (as opposed to financial) reasons why we prescribe generic aciclovir rather than the modern, more convenient, alternatives; or if there are disadvantages in not using the new products. Many trials have been performed around the world using these new antivirals, demonstrating their effect on acute infection, on suppressing recurrences and, most recently, on significantly cutting down transmission in discordant couples, those where one partner is positive for herpes and the other not. The new products have shown themselves to be very effective in all these circumstances: on 1 January, 2004, the *New England Journal of Medicine* (probably the most prestigious and influential medical journal in the world) published a paper showing a significant reduction in transmission of herpes in discordant couples who took valaciclovir compared with those taking placebo (inactive tablets). However, the cynics among us clinicians await, so far in vain, trials comparing the new products with the now out-of-patent aciclovir, rather than with sugar tablets.

Topical treatments in the form of creams or ointments are now available over the counter in the UK and are much advertised by their manufacturers. There is little evidence that they alter the course of an attack and are regarded by many as a waste of money. One trial showed that they diminished shedding of the herpes virus by all of half a day in an attack lasting over a week – not a brilliant result. No, simply keeping the sores moist (in contrast to old-fashioned advice to dry them) with petroleum jelly, Vaseline™, suffices for the short duration of most recurrences. The only time when topical aciclovir is effective and *must* be used is when there is herpetic keratitis involving the surface of the eye, thankfully very rare.

# What are the complications of herpes?

The main worry about herpes is its effect on the fetus in pregnancy or on the newborn baby. Debate still rages about the degree of risk and the likelihood of problems. There appear also to be significant differences between the figures from the USA and the UK, with many fewer problems in the UK.

On both sides of the Atlantic there is full agreement about the risk of transmission to the newborn baby if the mother suffers *a primary attack of herpes genitalis during the last few weeks of pregnancy*. This last sentence ends in italics to emphasize that the attack needs to be a primary (i.e. first ever) attack and it needs to be in the last few weeks of pregnancy. When this occurs, there is a real chance of the newborn catching herpes and suffering brain damage or death as a result. To put this into perspective in the UK, there are less than ten such cases per year out of 600 000 births. The risk is small.

Why is there not an equivalent risk with a *recurrent* attack? Probably it is a combination of factors but the most important is the transfer of antibodies from the mother to the baby across the placenta. Along with oxygen and nutrients the placenta also transmits a ready-made immune package full of antibodies to all the infections the mother has ever suffered from including this year's common cold, last year's 'flu and, most importantly, her HSV-1 or 2. This 'passive' immunity is quite enough to prevent any serious infection taking hold in the baby. Further, the number of virions (virus particles) is much, much less in a recurrent than in a primary attack.

Nonetheless there are some in the medical and nursing profession who perceive a large risk if a recurrence occurs around the time of birth. My advice to pregnant women with recurrent herpes in the 1980s and 1990s boiled down to a simple phrase: 'Don't tell your obstetrician'. Happily now gone are the days when women with herpes were examined at weekly intervals for their last six weeks of pregnancy and then subjected to a caesarean section at the first hint of an outbreak.

There have been several studies, largely from the USA, showing that, even when there are actual herpetic sores present on the vulva at the time of delivery, the baby does not develop infection. However, the widely held view remains that a caesarean section should be advised under these circumstances.

There used to be a belief that HSV infection was a predisposing factor in development of cancer of the cervix, perhaps because those who had more sexual partners were more likely to develop both herpes and cancer. It is now accepted that there is no connection and no extra risk.

Those who are HIV-positive and who also are infected with herpes (like everybody else, that means most) will get attacks that last longer and are rather less easy to get rid of. When this is the case, they may need to remain on long-term antiviral treatment. The best solution, however, is to have the HIV infection controlled with antiretroviral therapy (see Chapter 12) when the herpes should be no more problematic than for anyone else.

Some people become emotionally and psychologically involved with their condition, to the extent that their infection with genital herpes dominates their lives. It is easier to come to terms when it is realized that almost everybody else in the world has also got herpes (albeit more of them with labial than genital); that the chances of passing it on are low and can be even further diminished; that affordable treatment is readily available to virtually eliminate the possibility of a recurrence; and that they caught it from someone who, if they had known what they had done or at least understood how it happened, would have been mortified and, as likely as not, had not been unfaithful to them.

## Resources

Herpes Viruses Association: **www.herpes.org.uk**
**www.bashh.org/guidelines.htm**

# 8 Genital warts

Anogenital warts, sometimes called condylomas, are caused by certain types of human papilloma virus (HPV). Human papilloma viruses only affect humans but there are equivalent viruses for cats (feline), mice (murine) and cows (bovine), indeed for most animal species. There are many different subtypes of human papilloma viruses with HPV-6 and HPV-11 being the most common, found in 95 per cent of genital warts. These, along with HPV-42, 43 and 44, are 'low risk' (see cancer of the cervix, p. 96). There are more than ten 'intermediate risk' HPVs and a number of 'high risk' types including HPV-16, 18, 31, 33 and 45. I emphasize that only very few genital warts are of the high risk type.

## Have I got genital warts?

Probably not.

## Have I got anogenital HPV infection?

Quite possibly.

In November 2004, at a two-day conference in Cambridge devoted to the vulva, I asked one of the speakers, a world expert in the wart virus, whether I was correct to tell my female patients that, by the age of 25, up to 60 per cent of them would be infected with the virus that causes genital warts, human papilloma virus. 'No,' she said, 'up to 80 per cent would be a better estimate'.

In a funny way this figure, of perhaps four in five sexually active young women infected with wart virus, comes as a real relief to that minority who have gone on to develop clinical wart infection. To know that most of your contemporaries are also infected puts the condition into perspective. To also learn that, by the age of fifty, only a small number, less than 5 per cent, still carry the virus tells us that, in spite of the lack of a cure for HPV, we seem able to eradicate it ourselves as time goes by.

The figures for the prevalence of HPV infection in young men are less precise – it is almost certainly less common than in women but still probably over 50 per cent. The important thing is that most of those men or women, are unaware that they are infected and, unless they develop actual warts, will never know because detection of asymptomatic HPV infection is not an investigation routinely available.

So what is all the fuss about? Well, warts are a nuisance. They are unsightly, they don't feel right and they are embarrassing to have. Certain strains of HPV are also associated with cancerous changes. Most people know of the connection between wart virus and cancer of the cervix in women but these viruses can also (although less commonly) cause cancer of the penis, anus and rectum.

## Transmission of HPV

Genital warts are sexually transmitted. Like other STIs, almost all infections are passed on unwittingly by someone who is quite unaware of their infection. It is worth repeating: the large majority of HPV infections are present without any symptoms. Most people who have HPV infection do not know it.

### Case history

Mrs Beryl C, a 35-year-old career barrister, had been married for six years to another lawyer when she became pregnant. They had been in a monogamous relationship since she was 27 although they had both had previous sexual relationships. She was delighted at the news but mentioned at her first antenatal check-up that she had noticed some bumps on her labia which first appeared when she was about twelve weeks pregnant. The nurse at the GP's surgery had a quick look and told her that she had genital warts, that they were a sexually transmitted infection and that she should attend the local GUM clinic as soon as possible.

When I saw her she was very upset, having accused her husband of being unfaithful (he had vigorously denied an affair; she hadn't believed him) and was determined to obtain a termination of pregnancy, not wanting to bring a child into what was clearly a doomed, and soon to be sundered, relationship.

When I explained the figures for asymptomatic infection, told her that many of her colleagues and most of the pupils in her chambers were also infected with the wart virus and that she had probably had this infection for ten or fifteen years, she was somewhat mollified but was still suspicious at the coincidence of her pregnancy and the development of warts.

A further explanation of the effect of pregnancy on a mother's immuno-logical status – in simple terms the immune system becomes a little less aggressive so as not to harm the unborn child but this may allow warts to surface – eventually put her mind at rest. Both those who have had genital warts in the past and those without such a history (but with latent HPV infection) are prone to develop warts when they become pregnant. That's the bad news. The good news is that the warts tend to regress, even without treatment, after the baby is born. Mrs C insisted that her spouse attend the clinic and, with her new-found knowledge, was not too surprised that he turned out to have no evidence of warts at all.

The anogenital HPV types are usually confined to the nether regions. Occasionally, they may be found in the mouth or eyes and I once saw an Italian waiter with them in his ear but his lack of spoken English and mine of Italian meant that I never got an explanation. Rarely, a mother with genital infection can pass this on to her child during birth. The virus then may cause papillomatosis of the respiratory tract including laryngeal warts.

## What do warts look like?

Not all warts look the same. They can be flat or raised above the surrounding skin. If they are in a moist area, say between the vulva or under the foreskin, they have a softer surface like that of a raspberry, although thankfully smaller. These are known as exophytic warts. On skin exposed to the air, the outside becomes more like the top of a callus, with a harder, or 'keratinized', surface. These are known as sessile or papular warts. Warts can be as small as a pinhead up to the size of purple sprouting broccoli – the latter being rare!

All sorts of lumps or bumps in the genital area get confused with warts but there are two variations on normal human anatomy, that both turn up regularly in specialist clinics having been diagnosed as warts. The first, a quite common finding in men, are called Fordyce tubercles or 'pearly papules' and are to be seen as a ring of whitish bumps less than a millimetre across, encircling the glans just where it joins the shaft of the penis. Women's equivalent is vulval papillosis, little fleshy bumps, also smaller than a millimetre across, covering a postage stamp area or less, on the inside of the labia. Vulval papillosis and Fordyce tubercles are benign conditions that can be ignored. They do not go away if subjected to antiwart treatment.

Four other diagnoses can cause confusion. Sebaceous cysts are little enclosed pockets of secretion from the sebaceous glands in the skin and can occur almost anywhere. They can vary in size from a small ball-bearing up to a billiard ball or larger although, if they are in the genital region, they are likely to have been removed long before they reach that size. Folliculitis is, literally, an inflammation of a hair follicle. Any bit of skin that has hair follicles can develop folliculitis which, when it becomes badly infected, becomes a boil. Folliculitis and molluscum contagiosum (see page 120) are the two most likely diagnoses when lumps develop in the pubic area. Finally, near the entrance to the vagina and around the anus there are sometimes little extra bits of skin, known as skin tags.

Name any condition that causes raised lumps or bumps on the skin and, if it occurs in the anogenital area, it will be confused with warts. This is not the place for a list of these, suffice it to say that the six conditions described above will account for 95 per cent of all the 'warts' that turn out not to be warts.

## What treatments are available?

When we see wart infections in a GUM clinic, what is on offer is a 'cosmetic' exercise. That is to say, we do our best to eliminate visible and palpable warts but we cannot eradicate HPV. These are two important messages to grasp: that we can get rid of the troublesome lumps, in most cases fairly rapidly, and that irrespective of what the patient or we do, the virus infection will go, without outside intervention, as time goes by.

So, how do we set about getting rid of these visible warts? We can burn them off with electric current; freeze them to death; dissolve them with acid; put on substances that stop them, or rather the cells in which they are living, dividing; or try to stimulate a local immune reaction. Or we can bury a sixpenny piece (or a dime) in the garden and hope for the best.

Electrocautery was one of the earliest treatments and uses a metal prong through which an electric current is passed which literally burns off any material with which it comes into contact. The trouble is that it cannot distinguish between wart and normal flesh, so the operator needs a steady hand. As in a busy restaurant kitchen, you may need an extractor fan to disperse the fumes. Not many units still us this method.

Cryotherapy has been one of the most commonly used treatments in clinics for many years. In the old days freezing metal tips (cryoprobes made cold with nitrous oxide) were attached to a wart, using a little petroleum jelly, until the wart turned white with the cold. This was rather cumbersome and nowadays most operators use a 'gun' which has a nozzle through which a jet of liquid nitrogen is passed. The jet is pointed at the wart until, again, it turns white. The procedure is used for all the warts and may need to be repeated at weekly intervals, or occasionally more often until the warts are gone.

Given that one of the most reliable ways of preserving viruses and other micro-organisms is to pop them in a deep freezer where they can survive, frozen, for decades, freezing warts seems, initially, a slightly bizarre mode of treatment. However, freezing destroys the skin cell in which the virus resides. There are two schools of thought regarding the practicalities of using a liquid nitrogen spray. One says that it is necessary to freeze a small area around the wart, whereas the other suggests limiting the white area to the wart itself. There is no good evidence that either works better and, as freezing non-warty skin is painful, I prefer to concentrate on the wart alone.

Trichloroacetic acid (TCA) is a caustic alternative method which, like electrocautery, burns away the wart. As with electrocautery, however, the treatment cannot distinguish wart from normal skin and care is needed not to damage and leave scars. Putting a ring of Vaseline™ around the wart before treatment lessens the risk of burning from the acid.

Podophylline, an extract from the podophyllum plant, is an anti-mitotic agent, that is it stops cells dividing. If a cell is infected by HPV this lack of division means that the virus cannot reproduce and will die out. The standard clinic treatment for many years was an extract of podophylline, often 25 per cent by volume, made up in a brown substance, tincture of benzoin compound (TBC). The podophylline is not dissolved in the TBC, rather it is *suspended* which means that, if left standing for some time, the podophylline sinks to the bottom of the container. It should be shaken well before use. If not, the first patients simply have their warts painted brown while later patients are likely to have a very strong treatment applied.

A recent trial has shown that, if podophylline and cryotherapy are both used when a patient attends a clinic, the warts go more quickly than when only one or the other is used.

The final local treatment offered in clinic is 5-fluorocytosine, which has been used with some success particularly in warts that are difficult to get at, such as those just inside the urethra, intra-meatal, in the male.

For many years, the above treatments were all that were available and for those whose warts persisted, trailing up to the clinic for treatment week after week became a soul-destroying exercise. Two new methods of treatment, both of which can be used at home, have greatly eased the burden for those whose warts do not disappear quickly or readily.

The first new home treatment (it can be used in clinic as well) was an extract of podophylline, podophyllotoxin, which could be standardized to a particular strength and, as a cream or a lotion, was relatively easy for the patient to apply. Used three times weekly, for four weeks, it has a high success rate assuming that the warts are easy to get at (a mirror is supplied with some preparations).

The second home treatment is a totally novel approach which uses an immune-modulator, 5 per cent imiquimod, as a cream applied like podophyllotoxin, three times per week for four weeks. Imiquimod and podophylline, in whatever form, are contra-indicated in pregnancy because of a possible risk to the unborn child.

Both home treatments can cause quite severe soreness, particularly if spread on normal uninfected skin, so care is needed.

Before we realized how common HPV infection was and how it tends in nearly all cases to disappear of its own accord over time, we used to work hard trying to treat anal and rectal warts. Proctoscopy, passing a metal cylinder through the anus, was a regular and standard procedure in clinic to enable freezing or application of anti-wart substances. Most doctors now acknowledge that not only was this time-consuming procedure uncomfortable for the recipient but it made very little difference to the final outcome. These days many clinics only use a proctoscope if there is bleeding or warts are very large and are interfering with defecation.

Surgical treatment of warts, cutting them off under anaesthetic, is sometimes needed if they are inaccessible to local measures, particularly if they are just inside the anus or rectum. If it is possible, surgery for anogenital warts is best avoided as there is a high chance of recurrence within a few months of the operation.

## Cancer of the cervix

Up to 50 per cent of sexually active women will develop their HPV infection on the cervix, the neck of the womb. Some 10 per cent will have persisting infection of whom one-half may develop abnormalities. Perhaps one in five of those with abnormalities will need further treatment to prevent development of cancer.

However, cervical cancer is not evenly distributed throughout the population. The risk is increased in the poor, those who had early sexual intercourse, many sexual partners and many STIs. There is a slight extra risk in those who take the oral contraceptive but a particular added risk for smokers.

There have been several different ways of classifying these cervical abnormalities. Dysplasia or dyskaryosis are the terms used to describe the abnormal changes on cervical cytology samples (cervical smear test). Koilocytosis is the term used to describe wart infection of the cervix when it shows up on cytology. Squamous intraepithelial lesions (SIL), is replacing cervical intraepithelial neoplasia (CIN) as a way of describing the changes that take place in a biopsy sample, when the tissue of the cervix is examined under the microscope. Similar alterations in wart-infected tissue can affect the penis (PIN), the vulva (VIN) and the anus (AIN). All these changes, when they become severe, are tending towards the diagnosis without actually being cancer. Luckily, there are highly effective treatments that cure.

The screening system of cervical smear tests has been one of the most successful public health measures over the past thirty years and has been shown to have radically reduced the number of cases of cancer of the cervix. However, there are pitfalls if the tests are performed on very young women. There are often suspicious-looking findings in the smear tests of those under 20 that do not mean that early cancerous changes are occurring. Many clinicians believe it is better not to perform cervical cytology until after women are at least 21.

The current recommendations for cervical cytology in the UK suggest repeating every three years. Many people believe this could be extended to every five years. There are developments attempting to combine cytology with identification of any HPV that is present, at the same time. If and when this becomes available, it will be possible to reassure most of those who have low risk types of HPV that they are very unlikely to go on to develop cancer.

Colposcopy is a procedure that enables the operator, usually the doctor, to examine the surface of the cervix under magnification. This can produce an image from two to sixty times normal and enables abnormalities to be identified with greater accuracy. Acetic acid (the active ingredient in vinegar) is applied to the surface of the cervix and can highlight abnormal cells which turn a whitish colour. If there are areas that need further investigation, a biopsy can be taken and, if and when the laboratory shows suspicious cells, it is a simple matter to remove the offending tissue by freezing, burning or cutting off, or a combination of these.

## Vaccines against HPV

The wart virus has a different effect on the immune system from that of other viruses which may explain why it is so persistent. While other viruses, under normal circumstances, kill the cells they have infected, the wart virus has chosen a cell that is destined to die anyway in a short time: the skin cell. Keratinocytes make their way towards the surface of normal skin and, when they reach the surface, slough off as dead skin. As this is a normal process, there is none of the inflammation which would accompany the killing of other cells by a virus. If there is no inflammation, this means no stimulation of an immune response by the body.

A recent exciting development, reported in the *Lancet* in early 2005, suggests success with a new vaccine against HPV. Over 500 women aged between 16 and 23, in the USA, Brazil and Europe, were either given a vaccine against four of the HPV types, or a placebo. The four HPVs were 6 and 11, the common, 'low risk' varieties, and 16 and 18, both 'high risk' and responsible for 70 per cent of all cervical cancer. The trial was double-blind which means that neither the doctors nor the women knew whether they had been given vaccine or placebo. The women in the trial were followed up for two and a half years at the end of which time, three had developed warts and three CIN, the pre-cancerous changes. Each one of these six women was in the placebo group, that is they had not received the active vaccine.

It will be a year or two before vaccines such as this one (and there are others being developed with equally encouraging early results) are on the market but one can foresee a time when all young girls are vaccinated against HPV before they become sexually active, just as they are against rubella. If all goes well, tomorrow's generation of women will miss out on the tedium of regular smear tests, never suffer from genital warts and, most importantly of all, be free of the risk of cervical cancer in all but the rarest of cases.

## Resources

www.bashh.org/guidelines.htm

# 9 Syphilis and related diseases

## Historical aspects

Syphilis, with gonorrhoea, is one of the oldest venereal diseases and as such has a history that goes back possibly to biblical times, although some people believe the disease to be more recent, in Europe at least. The 'pre-Columbian' school uses evidence from ancient bones found in Europe and North Africa to argue that syphilis was around in pre-Christian days.

There are many references in the Old Testament to conditions with signs and symptoms that would do well for syphilis. In Deuteronomy, those who disobeyed the laws were threatened by Moses with the 'Botch of Egypt' which, after scabs and emerods, progressed to madness, blindness and astonishment of heart. One translation, from Psalms, threatens 'you will be smitten with the Egyptian dermatitis, characterized by swellings, dry crusts and ulcers . . . and the Lord shall smite you in the knees, and in the legs, with a sore botch that cannot be healed from the sole of thy foot to the top of thy head'. Ouch!

The visiting of the iniquity of their fathers on succeeding generations in the Third Commandment and the banning of 'he that hath a flat nose' and '. . . the fathers have eaten a sour grape and the children's teeth are set on edge', are all suggestive of congenital syphilis.

Those who subscribe to a more modern origin for syphilis rely on Columbus's (or more probably his crew's) role in the syphilis epidemic that engulfed Europe at the end of the fifteenth century. The 'Columbian' school believes that syphilis was endemic in North America and was brought back to Barcelona in 1493 after Columbus's first expedition. Certainly a contemporary physician, Dr Diza de Isla wrote of treating some of the crew for 'bubas' and the 'serpentine disease', although no reference is made to a sore botch. The siege of Naples took place the following year when Charles VIII of France crossed the Alps into Italy. Some, presumably infected, Spaniards joined his forces as mercenaries. By the spring of 1495 such a dreadful plague had broken out among those involved in the siege that it collapsed and a disorganized retreat ensued.

As they made their way home, the various nationalities spread syphilis which, following the example of the 'botch of Egypt', was usually blamed on a foreign enemy. The English called it the French disease; the French called it the Italian disease; the Italians, ever indecisive, called it the French disease *and* the Spanish disease; while the Spanish called it the disease of Hispaniola (Haiti), an island that, nearly 500 years later, was again suggested as a trans-Atlantic staging post for a sexually transmitted infection (Chapter 11). Whether or not any particular nation was at fault, the French aggressors, perhaps appropriately, were eventually blamed, because syphilis was generally referred to in later centuries as the morbus gallicus, the Latin for French disease.

Syphilis, 'the pox', became widespread in Europe and carried considerable social stigma, as this extract from the Manchester Quarter Sessions of 1651 illustrates:

> ...to the right worshipful Justices of the Peace and quorum for the County pallatyne of Lancaster
>
> Right worshipfulls
>
> This may be to acqaynt you that there is a pore yong women in oure Towne of Asston-undrlyne infected with a filthy deceassd called the French poxe and shee saith shee was defiled by one Henry Heyworth a maryed man, but soe it is the report of that dessease occasioneth neighbours to deny hir harbour and shee is enforced to lye in the streetes and in great danger to bee starved, I do humbly intreate your worshipps to take it into your consideration and to grant your Order that the pore woman may be provyded for to prevent starveing, either upon the parrish charges, or upon the Costs of the said Heyworth whom she saith hath spoiled hir, whether yiur worshipps shall think fitt

The court was generous, while not mincing its words, in its judgement '... to erect some small cottage or Cabin for her in regard to her lothesomenes'.

## Are there many cases today?

Syphilis in the UK, like gonorrhoea, peaked at the end of the Second World War and the numbers then dropped precipitously to the mid-1950s. The two diseases then diverged, gonorrhoea increasing greatly while syphilis numbers remained low until almost the end of the twentieth century and were confined, apart from occasional imported cases, to homosexual men. In 1997 there was an outbreak of syphilis among heterosexuals in Bristol associated with commercial sex work and crack cocaine use. This was followed by similar outbreaks in Newcastle, Edinburgh, Glasgow, Nottingham and Northern Ireland. Outbreaks in Scotland and in Manchester, Brighton and London have been largely among men who have sex with men (MSM) but have recently included an increasing number of heterosexual cases. Between April 2001 and September 2004, there were 1910 cases of syphilis in London, 1276 in MSM, 383 in heterosexual men and 237 in women.

Disturbingly, more than 50 per cent of MSM with syphilis were also HIV-positive. The epidemic is taking place in an increasing culture of unsafe sex particularly with partners whose HIV status is unknown. Casual sexual partners are now being acquired via internet chat rooms in addition to the 'traditional' venues such as saunas, clubs and cruising grounds.

There was a volcanic increase in cases of syphilis following the social and political changes in the old USSR in the early 1990s. This epidemic crossed Russia and headed towards the Baltic States and was initially mainly heterosexually driven although there is evidence that infections among MSM are now increasing.

## What causes syphilis?

Syphilis is caused by a bacterium, *Treponema pallidum*, a thin, spiral, flexible micro-organism which makes its way with a combination of corkscrew and bending movements. It has a capacity to invade just about every part of the body and, in the days before antibiotics, the ravages of syphilis were common, with many people suffering from the late stages of the infection, which might involve the nervous system and the heart and blood vessels. The treponeme needs a small cut or abrasion in the skin before it can gain entry and cause infection. This is thought to be one of the reasons for the disease being more common among male homosexuals, as anal intercourse is more traumatic than vaginal sex and more likely to cause skin tears.

Syphilis is seen in two forms – acquired and congenital. The acquired form of the disease is almost invariably the result of sexual activity with an infected person, while congenital syphilis, as its name implies, is passed on passively while the developing fetus is *in utero*.

## How is it diagnosed?

In early infectious syphilis, the treponeme can be found in the primary sore and in the secondary rash and, using a special GUM clinic microscope, it is possible to identify it by looking at a little fluid squeezed from the lesions. This is called a dark-ground or dark-field examination and, if positive, gives a definitive diagnosis. This test has to be performed very carefully and is not always successful. Therefore, a great reliance is placed on blood tests, which become positive early in the infection.

The blood tests measure the presence of antibodies to syphilis in the blood. Some of these tests, exemplified by the Venereal Disease Research Laboratories (VDRL) test (another one called the RPR works in a similar fashion), are useful because they give a clue as to whether the syphilis is still active, depending on how strongly positive the test is. Others, such as the Treponema Pallidum Haemagglutination Test (TPHA), Fluorescent Treponemal Antibody-Absorption Test (FTA) or Enzyme Immunoassay (EIA) remain positive forever following infection, even after successful treatment. It must be remembered that these continuing positive blood tests do *not* suggest that the disease is still active, any more than a positive blood test for rubella or measles means anything more than that the person has had the infection in the past.

## What are the symptoms and stages of acquired syphilis?

Not for nothing was syphilis known to physicians of the pre-antibiotic era as the 'great imitator'. In its earliest stage, soon after infection, the diagnosis may be relatively easy but thereafter, from the rash of secondary syphilis to the complications involving the nervous and cardiovascular systems, the diagnosis will be difficult to make, particularly as the afflicted person is likely to go to any specialist rather than one who knows about sexually transmitted infections.

In the first stage of syphilis there is a sore known as the primary chancre which appears between one and twelve weeks after infection, although most usually at between two and four weeks. By the time the, usually solitary, chancre appears the treponeme has already travelled to the nearby lymph nodes where it has multiplied considerably, so application of antiseptics or antibiotic creams will have no effect on the disease. The sore is not usually painful and has a hard floor which may feel like a small button just below the skin surface. It varies between barely visible to the size of a small fingernail. It has an evil appearance but is almost always completely pain-less, as are the swollen lymph glands nearby.

The chancre is most often found on the penis where it is hard to miss. It is not so obvious in women, when on the vulva, in the vagina, or even on the cervix; or in either sex if it is on or around the anus. This primary sore is sometimes found on the lips, nipples, tongue or other sites. One particularly unfortunate occurrence is at the base of the penis, the so-called 'condom chancre'. In such cases proper precautions have been taken but a sore on the vulva, say, has come into contact with that lower part of the unlucky individual's penis not covered by the condom.

The primary sore of syphilis is followed some six to eight weeks later by the secondary stage. The primary sore is still present in perhaps one-third of cases.

By the time the secondary stage has started, the bacterium has spread throughout the body. Because it is most easy to see, it is popularly believed that the skin rash, which occurs in three-quarters of people, is the most important affliction. However, if the treponeme is looked for, it can be found affecting all the parts of the body, from the liver to the lungs and the brain to the bones. People with secondary syphilis feel generally unwell with fever, aches and pains and loss of appetite. In one-half there will be generalized enlargement of the lymph glands.

## Case history

Philip H, a 35-year-old music arranger was seen at the ear, nose and throat department of a Midlands hospital with ringing in his ears. This tinnitus is a symptom of several medical conditions, ranging from excess wax to middle ear infection or inflammation of the auditory nerve. Had a sexual history been taken at the time of his first visit, it would have emerged that, although he had a long-lasting and stable sexual relationship with one person, his partner was promiscuous and had had a number of casual sexual partners over the preceding year. As it was, all manner of sophisticated tests failed to reveal the cause of his tinnitus. Poor Philip was particularly bothered because he had perfect pitch and the ringing in his ears was a quarter tone below middle C and therefore 'out of tune'.

When he was seen in the GUM clinic, after blood tests for syphilis, taken as a last resort, had turned out strongly positive, he remembered having had a sore on his penis some five months earlier but had not bothered with it as it was not painful and had gone away after a couple of weeks. He had not noticed any skin rash and was surprised to be told that his symptom was a direct result of syphilis affecting the auditory nerve. Within one week of his first penicillin injection the ringing was gone and he was able to resume work.

This particular complication is, of course, rare but there is some evidence of involvement of the central nervous system in perhaps 20 per cent of cases of secondary syphilis although there may be nothing more than a slight headache to show for it. The eyes, liver, joints and bones can all be involved but will all be difficult to diagnose without the coincidental and helpful skin and mucous membrane signs.

After a period of some weeks the rash and any other complications of secondary syphilis will go of their own accord and the disease enters its early latent stage. This lasts until the end of the second year after initial infection and is not characterized by any signs or symptoms although infectious bacteria are still present in the tissues. Rarely, there is a recurrence of the secondary stage when the rash or other complications return for a short while. Relapse of infection can occur in some cases that have been treated. This may result from inadequate treatment and is more common in those who were treated late in the secondary stage. It is for this reason that patients are followed up for two years after treatment. It should be said that reinfection is rather more common than relapse as a cause of reappearance of active syphilis.

The late latent stage of syphilitic infection starts at the end of year two and heralds a period when there is virtually no chance of the infection being passed on. Many who have reached this stage can look forward to no further trouble from their infection and will die of old age or an unrelated condition. Those in whom syphilis does continue to be active, progress to late syphilis.

The lesion in tertiary syphilis is known as the gumma. A gumma results from blockage of small arteries and can cause skin lesions or sometimes lumps or nodules under the skin. Painless ulcers can be found in the mouth or on the palate and may spread to involve the underlying bone. The tongue, bones, muscles and internal organs can all be involved by gummatous change. These later changes of syphilis are very, very uncommon in the Western world today.

Perhaps 10 per cent of patients with late, untreated syphilis will go on to develop cardiovascular syphilis with disease of the heart and major blood vessels. The first of three important complications is aortic regurgitation, where some of the blood pumped from the heart is allowed to flow backwards to the heart rather than passing on round the circulation. This happens because the valve where the large main blood vessel, the aorta, leaves the heart becomes faulty. This puts a huge strain on the heart muscle which will eventually fail.

The second complication occurs when the syphilitic process affects the opening of the coronary arteries. These become narrowed which may lead to angina, if not a heart attack. The third cardiovascular complication is the development of aneurysms in the wall of the aorta or other major blood vessels. An aneurysm is a swelling or dilatation caused by weakness in the wall of a blood vessel.

Involvement of the nervous system by the syphilitic process is known as neurosyphilis. The first of two main categories is general paralysis of the insane (GPI), in which there is progressive deterioration in brain function. This is often noticed only by close friends or relatives but not by the person themselves. The memory is lost and judgement is impaired. The classical progression is then to delusions of grandeur with absurd claims of past and present achievements. More commonly there is a gradually increasing dementia with depression. There is a physical decline with fits, incontinence, difficulty with speech and a degree of spastic paralysis.

If the spinal cord, rather than the brain, is involved the condition is known as tabes dorsalis. The main features of tabes are an inability to balance when the eyes are shut, numbness and 'tingling' sensations and 'lightning pains', which are sharp, shooting pains, usually in the lower limbs which may come and go in a short time or last for several days. Bowel and bladder function can become disturbed and there may be damage to the sacral nerves which supply the genitalia, leading to sexual anaesthesia in women and impotence in men. Because the sensory (feeling) nerves are involved, minor damage to joints is not noticed and severe arthritis eventually develops. Optic atrophy gradually leading to blindness complicates 20 per cent of cases of tabes.

## Congenital syphilis

Syphilis can be passed on to the unborn fetus if the mother is infected and has *Treponema pallidum* circulating in her blood stream. The father cannot directly infect the fetus without first infecting the mother. The longer the mother has had syphilis, the lower the risk of it being passed on to her unborn child and the less severe will be the congenital syphilis if it *is* passed on. Thus a woman with early infectious syphilis is likely either to miscarry or give birth to a stillborn child. If she has early latent syphilis there is a 20 per cent chance that the child will be unaffected. This figure rises to 70 per cent unaffected if the mother has late syphilis.

In most countries when a woman becomes pregnant her blood is tested for syphilis. And this one measure is responsible for the extreme rarity of young cases of congenital syphilis. Of course the figures vary enormously between different countries. Worldwide there are an estimated 1 million children born with congenital syphilis each year and 10 per cent of pregnant women in Africa are said to be infected with syphilis. By contrast, in the seven years between 1997 and 2003, there were fewer than fifteen admissions for congenital syphilis in children under ten years of age in the UK.

Congenital syphilis is arbitrarily divided into early and late stages with the dividing line at two years of age. There is no primary stage in congenital syphilis just as in adult syphilis acquired from a blood transfusion or a needlestick injury.

The affected baby may be quite normal at birth or may have the neonatal equivalent of the secondary stage with rash and enlarged lymph nodes. The mucous membrane lesions lead to 'snuffles' with a nasal discharge, classically 'teeming' with treponemes. This is highly infectious to anyone who comes into contact, apart from the mother (who, obviously, already has the disease and so cannot catch it). There may also be liver, bone and eye involvement with, occasionally, meningitis.

In some cases of late congenital syphilis it may be difficult to tell whether the infection is congenital or acquired. The most common manifestation is interstitial keratitis, a clouding of the cornea in front of the eye. Late neurological complications can occur, equivalent to those in late acquired syphilis but for some reason, the cardiovascular complications are virtually never seen.

Certain so-called 'stigmata' may be seen in congenital syphilis – these are the residual scars and deformities of early infection. These are not invariable and many with congenital syphilis have only abnormal blood tests to show for their infection. However there may be abnormalities of the teeth, Hutchinson's teeth, and the facial appearance may be diagnostic if the nasal infection was severe. The bridge of the nose is depressed looking a little like a saddle and the upper jaw may be small compared with the lower. This gives a typical 'bulldog' appearance. Small scars at the corner of the mouth are known as rhagades.

## What is the treatment?

The treponeme is sensitive to a variety of antibiotics and it was thought that the fall in number of cases after the war might be due to 'chance' treatment as people were given penicillin or tetracycline for unrelated problems, such as inflammation of the bladder (cystitis) or chest infections. However, before penicillin was discovered (in the 1930s), an extraordinary succession of treatments waxed and waned over the centuries, many of them appearing to work well simply because the signs and symptoms of early infectious syphilis, the chancre and rash, got better of their own accord in a matter of months or weeks.

## Evolution of treatment

Guy de Chauliac's treatment for scabies, invented in 1363, contained, among other things, wild delphinium, gum-resin, lead oxide, old pig's fat and one-ninth part mercury. When the morbus gallicus, the 'French disease', surfaced at the end of the next century, this unction was used extensively in its treatment, apparently with good (but, rarely curative) effect. The physicians of the day as well as 'Butchers, sow-gelders, farriers and itinerant mountebanks', were aware of the ointment's dangers (perhaps a combination of the lead and the mercury) which included belly-ache, excess salivation and caused the teeth to fall out. The problem lay in the fact that the curative dose of the mercury was very close to the lethal dose.

Briefly in the sixteenth century, mercury was supplanted by a bark extract, *Guaiacum*. In 1519, the poet Von Hutten wrote of the blessed relief of this new product when compared with the tortures of mercury treatment and a contemporary, Fracastorius, wrote a poem in which the shepherd, Syphilis, was cured by guaiacum. These two early advertisements did wonders for the product until Von Hutten died of late syphilis aged 35, in spite of his 'cure'. When Barbarossa, an Algerian pirate, learnt in 1537 that Francis I of France had acquired syphilis, he sent the King a present of pills containing, among other things, mercury. The royal endorsement meant that this poison again became the mainstay of treatment.

In 1732 Thomas Dover published a treatise in which he advocated the use of metallic mercury for a variety of medical complaints pointing out that, taken in this form, it did not have the side-effects of mercury compounds. Metallic mercury was not absorbed and was voided naturally in the faeces. Many was the tale of finding globules of mercury in people's shoes and in one story, a lady's partner at a fine ball thought she had dropped her pearls only to find, greatly to his consternation and her confusion, that they were the ubiquitous globules of mercury.

The first really viable alternatives to mercury arrived in the early twentieth century when arsenic compounds, particularly salvarsan, started to be used. Malarial treatment followed by the 'fever' box (which mimicked the high temperature but without the malaria) and injections of bismuth into the buttocks were the last of a succession of unconventional and doubtful cures before penicillin became generally available after the Second World War.

## Modern treatment of syphilis

Penicillin, which revolutionized the treatment of syphilis when it was introduced, has remained the mainstay of management. The treponeme, unlike the gonococcus, has shown no sign of developing resistance to penicillin or any other antibiotics. When it was first used, penicillin was given by daily injections and this sort of regimen continued into the 1980s in certain clinics. This treatment is highly effective but smacks of a rather punitive approach to the patient, now that long-acting forms of penicillin have become available which can be given weekly rather than daily. Having said that, there is evidence that benzathine penicillin, the longer lasting form, does not penetrate the cerebro-spinal fluid (CSF) very well and doubts have been cast on its efficacy when there is involvement of the central nervous system. Other antibiotics including the tetracyclines and macrolides can be used when there is penicillin allergy.

The Jarisch-Herxheimer reaction, usually shortened to the 'Herxheimer' reaction, follows the initial treatment of syphilis in a number of cases. It is thought to be due to the break-up of dying treponemes which release inflammatory substances both locally and into the bloodstream. It is characterized by a 'flu-like illness lasting 12–24 hours with headache, aches and pains in muscles and joints, and fever. It occurs most frequently and least dangerously in early syphilis, perhaps in 50 per cent of cases. In late syphilis it is rare but, when it occurs, it can have catastrophic results. This is because the local inflammation that happens can result in local swelling resulting in blockage. Thus a Herxheimer reaction involving the opening to the coronary arteries can close them sufficiently to cause a heart attack. I have seen a person develop paralysis of both legs due to blockage of the small arteries supplying the spinal cord following his first penicillin injection. Luckily in this case full function returned within three days. Anti-inflammatory drugs such as steroids may be given in the hope of preventing such occurrences.

## Syphilis and HIV infection

The predominance of MSM among those with syphilis in Western countries has been mentioned and it is therefore no surprise to that HIV infection is also commonly found at the same time as syphilis. What is not clear is why HIV-positive persons are over-represented among MSM with syphilis. It may be that it is simply because both infections are found with unsafe sexual practices or a result of active syphilis (as with other genital ulcer diseases like herpes and chancroid) making transmission of HIV more likely. Or, it may be that having HIV makes the transmission of syphilis more likely. Whatever the reason, 30–40 per cent of MSM with syphilis were HIV-positive in Brighton and Amsterdam, 50 per cent in Paris and Berlin, and 60 per cent in London.

# Does HIV infection alter syphilis?

It has been suggested that early syphilis presents in a different way when there is concurrent HIV infection. The primary chancre is usually (two-thirds of cases) a single ulcer; in HIV infection two-thirds have multiple ulcers. It also seems that the primary chancre remains present in the secondary stage more frequently (at 45 per cent, three times more often). There have been suggestions that involvement of the nervous system is more common, particularly with eye complications, and that the disease in general progresses more rapidly, but these tend to be anecdotal (see Chapter 2), rather than comparative, reports.

There have also been anecdotes of cases of secondary syphilis with totally negative blood tests for syphilis. More data are needed. There are very few studies, or even anecdotes, about late syphilis in HIV-positive individuals. The standard treatment, in amount and length, seems to work with equal efficiency irrespective of HIV status.

# Tropical treponematoses

There are four conditions caused by bacteria seemingly identical to *Treponema pallidum* but which run courses quite different from syphilis. They cause problems not by the disease they produce (which is usually of negligible clinical significance) but because infection with them gives blood test results identical to those found in syphilis. Some of these infections go through similar stages and periods of latency but why these occur, sometimes co-existing with syphilis, yet have such different clinical outcomes, is not known.

Yaws, occurring in tropical climates, used to be endemic in parts of Africa, South America, Indonesia, Australia and the West Indies. The bacterium in yaws is called *Treponema pertenue* but the different name does not make it distinguishable from *Treponema pallidum*. It is not sexually transmitted (apart from the fact that, like chicken pox or influenza, it could be) and is usually acquired in early childhood by innocent contact with another infected child. The primary sore, known as the 'mother yaw', often occurs on the leg and, like the chancre in syphilis, is painless. There may follow a secondary stage with rash and, very rarely, late stages including gangosa, a mutilating destructive process involving the nose and palate. Even more rarely, involvement of the central nervous system is seen. It is often impossible, when seeing someone from an endemic area with positive serological tests for syphilis (STS), to know whether these are due to yaws or syphilis so it is customary to treat with an 'insurance' injection of penicillin.

Bejel, known as 'loath' and 'firzal' in the Middle East and 'dichuchwa' in Botswana can also present with skin and mucous membrane lesions and sometimes goes on to involve the larynx and bones. Like yaws, most infections occur in childhood, and it is said that adults who have escaped infection when young can be infected by their own children, a reversal of roles from congenital syphilis. Late complications do not occur and, as with yaws, penicillin is the treatment of choice.

Pinta, found in Central and South America, is the least damaging of the treponematoses and like yaws and bejel, is often acquired in childhood. The primary sore, the pintid, often appears on the legs and is followed by a secondary stage. *Treponema careatum*, the cause of pinta, is, like *T. pertenue*, indistinguishable from *T. pallidum*.

Endemic syphilis occurs when so many people in a community have syphilis that transmission occurs regularly by non-sexual contact. Such a situation existed in Bosnia around the time of the Second World War. Primary infection occurs in children and infants and the way the disease progresses is the same as in adult infection but, obviously, happens at a younger age. Congenital syphilis is rare in these circumstances because, by the time women get to child-bearing age, the disease has entered the late stage when transmission to the fetus is less likely.

Following an intensive campaign by the World Health Organization, in which everyone at possible risk was given penicillin, endemic syphilis was eradicated in that part of what was then Yugoslavia.

## Resources

www.bashh.org/guidelines.htm

# 10 Tropical and other infections

This chapter contains a hotch-potch of different conditions, none of which deserves a chapter all to itself but each of which is important in its own way, particularly if you've caught it or think you have. There are three tropical diseases, lymphogranuloma venereum (LGV), chancroid and donovanosis. None of these has been at all common in Western Europe for many decades until a recent outbreak of LGV in MSM, most of whom are HIV-positive. Then there are the two infestations, 'crabs' and scabies. A number of diarrhoea-causing infections referred to, rather inaccurately, as 'gay bowel' syndrome and, finally, a variety of conditions caused by viruses. There is a skin condition molluscum contagiosum; cytomegalovirus which can be sexually transmitted and poses problems in immunocompromised individuals; and the three viruses associated with hepatitis, A, B and C.

## Lymphogranuloma venereum (LGV)

LGV is caused by certain subtypes of *Chlamydia trachomatis*, the 'L' varieties (see Chapter 5). Until recently, the only cases seen in the UK were imported having been acquired in foreign parts, sub-Saharan Africa, South America and South-East Asia being the most likely areas. Since 2003 an increasing number of infections have been seen in HIV-positive homosexual men with outbreaks in Belgium, Holland, France and the UK.

## What does LGV do?

The incubation period is usually between one and three weeks and the first sign is a small, transient sore which is so insignificant that male patients miss it in 50 per cent of cases. Because this little ulcer will be in the vagina or on the labia, in women it is rarely noticed at all. Likewise an early rectal sore will be missed in MSM. After a further period of one to four weeks there will be enlargement of the lymph glands in the groin, the inguinal nodes, causing a swelling known as a bubo. This is a painful and progressive usually one-sided condition which, if untreated, will turn into large abscesses that can break down and discharge pus. The enlarged glands group into two sausage-shaped collections with a noticeable demarcation between them known as the 'sign of the groove'.

Women may not develop as marked a bubo as men with penile infection. Similarly if the primary infection is confined to the rectum, there may be no inguinal swelling at all because the lymph drainage is to lymph glands within the abdominal cavity rather than to the groin. This may lead to backache and occasionally, if the discomfort is right-sided, the pain may be mistaken for appendicitis. Their relative lack of symptoms probably explains why late complications are more common and more serious in women.

As its name implies, LGV affects the lymph glands and lymphatic channels which, when blocked, allow a build-up of fluid in the tissues, with swelling known as chronic lymphatic oedema. If untreated this swelling becomes permanent and is known as elephantiasis. In women the vulva become grossly enlarged, 'esthiomene', with swelling extending from the clitoris to the anus. A rare if intriguing complication of lymphoedema of the penis is the 'saxophone penis'.

Late complications of LGV, collectively called anorectal syndrome, are more common in women than men and involve the lower bowel with fistulas, such as between the rectum or bladder and the vagina, and stricture. Cancer of the lower bowel has been described as a rare complication. These complications have been recognized in homosexual men for many years but may increase in numbers in the future.

## Case history

Michel J was a 37-year-old single film editor who lived in Lille and whose job regularly took him to many different European countries. He had an 'open' relationship with Claude, his long-term partner, which allowed casual relationships with other men but these did not involve any penetrative sex, being limited to oral sex, fellatio. They had both tested negative for HIV infection two years previously. For a week Michel had stomach cramps with a little diarrhoea which he put down to food poisoning but when he noticed fresh blood on his underwear he became worried and consulted his family doctor.

He was reassured and prescribed some diarrhoea medicine but five days later his cramps became severe enough to take him to the local hospital. There he was noted to have a high fever and was admitted for observation in case he had an acute intestinal condition. The professor of gastroenterology was brought in and he advised a biopsy. Michel was asked about any family history of bowel conditions and also asked about recent travel. He had been in Amsterdam six weeks previously but this was at least a month before his symptoms had appeared. The biopsy report showed changes compatible with Crohn's disease, an inflammation of the bowel, and treatment was started for that.

A chance meeting with the local dermato-venereologist alerted the professor to the possibility of LGV and a sample from the bowel tested positive for an 'L' serovar of chlamydia confirming the diagnosis. Unfortunately an HIV test was also positive and it appeared that Michel had picked up both infections at a gay club in Amsterdam where, although no penile penetration took place, he had allowed insertion of a hand into his rectum, 'fisting', which can damage the delicate skin of the anus giving an ideal opportunity for infection to be transmitted. Michel subsequently also tested positive for hepatitis C bringing the total of infections picked up in one night to three.

## How is LGV diagnosed and treated?

The differential clinical diagnosis of early LGV includes any of the infections that cause genital ulceration including syphilis, chancroid and donovanosis. However, genital herpes is probably the most likely condition with which it could be confused. The laboratory tests that detect the NSU strains of *Chlamydia trachomatis* will also pick up LGV, a tentative diagnosis that can be confirmed in a specialist laboratory. A rising level of antibodies to LGV in the blood is suggestive of the diagnosis.

Not surprisingly, the treatment of LGV uses the same antibiotics as for NSU, the tetracyclines and macrolides like erythromycin, although the course is longer, usually lasting for two to three weeks.

## Chancroid

Also called 'soft sore', 'soft chancre' and 'ulcus molle', chancroid is a tropical disease which, like LGV, is usually only seen in Western Europe or North America when it has been imported. The main endemic areas are South and East Africa, India and Caribbean countries. Its name implies clinical features similar to the primary sore of syphilis, the chancre, but in reality it bears little resemblance. Unlike the classical chancre, the ulceration in chancroid is usually painful, the sores are multiple and the lesions are soft, not indurated and hard, as in syphilis.

The bacterium responsible is called *Haemophilus ducreyi* and it is fastidious, an adjective applied to bacteria that microbiologists find difficult to culture in the laboratory, and it is also hard to identify from the sores themselves using a microscope. This, coupled with its comparative rarity in the Western world, has led some cynical physicians to doubt its very existence as a separate entity. This view is lent some support by the extraordinary variety of clinical descriptions of the sores themselves. The ulcers can be dwarf, giant, transient, phagedenic (as in oeso*phagus*, eating flesh), follicular, papular, indeed almost any dermatological description will have been applied to chancroid at some point.

In spite of the foregoing, chancroid *is* a discrete clinical entity but the diagnosis may be mistaken when it is made in an area where the disease is rare. It used to be described as a disease of the 'socially unenlightened and economically unfortunate' which, if so, would make it unique among sexually transmitted diseases as a respecter of social class.

## What does chancroid do?

The spots or sores develop, usually on the penis (men outnumber women five to one), within seven days of infection. These are acutely painful and, in women, the discomfort is increased by urine running over the infected areas, an external dysuria. As with LGV the infection spreads to the nearby inguinal lymph nodes in the groin and a bubo may form. If untreated this swelling eventually breaks down and discharges pus. The famous 'groove sign', thought only to be found with LGV, can occur with chancroid as well. In parts of the world where chancroid is common it is an important co-factor in HIV transmission.

## How is chancroid diagnosed and treated?

One can be certain of the diagnosis when the actual bacterium is cultured in the laboratory although it is not that uncommon to find that other pathogens, such as herpes genitalis, are present at the same time.

Many groups of antibiotics including the macrolides, quinolones and cephalosporins work against *Haemophilus ducreyi* although, as with gonorrhoea, less sensitive strains are being now seen more frequently than ever.

## Donovanosis (granuloma inguinale)

Called *Donovania granulomatis* in the first edition, rapidly superseded by *Calymmatobacterium granulomatis* and next, and currently, *Klebsiella granulomatis*, the organism that causes donovanosis seems to give as much trouble to microbiological taxonomists as does to the clinicians who have to diagnose and treat it. This condition occurs in small pockets around the world, in southern Africa, parts of aboriginal Australia, Papua New Guinea, Brazil, China and the Caribbean. As with the previous two conditions, cases in Europe or North America will have been imported from an endemic region.

This is a fairly uninfectious organism and to catch it you need a break in normal skin. It is more common in darker skinned individuals and only some 50 per cent of sexual partners end up infected, even after prolonged exposure. Although it is not certain, the fact that the lesions are found largely in the anogenital area suggests that it is mostly sexually transmitted.

## What does it do?

The incubation period seems to have a wide range, from a few days to two months. It starts as a small papule or spot which ulcerates and spreads outwards leaving a raised, velvety reddened area that bleeds easily. It may spread to involve the perineum, thighs and buttocks and, although it does not provoke enlargement of the inguinal lymph glands like chancroid and LGV, there may be small nodules under the skin, pseudo-buboes. The area involved enlarges slowly over a period of months if not years. If there is infection of the cervix, it may look very much like a carcinoma. It is important to prevent transmission to the baby at childbirth and caesarean section may be needed if the cervix is involved by the infection.

Treatment is with broad-spectrum antibiotics but some resistance has been noted to tetracyclines. The newer macrolide, azithromycin, has been used with success. Because of its slow progression and low infectivity, it should be possible to eradicate completely and such control programmes are being tried in some parts of the world.

## The infestations

There are many arthropods associated with human disease, ranging from the larvae of certain flies such as the Congo maggot which eats away at human flesh, to the scorpion whose sting causes serious illness and even sometimes death in children. Fleas, ticks and spiders of various kinds are associated with disease either directly as a result of their bites or because they act as vectors of infections such as typhus or sleeping sickness. While it would be rash to claim that cochliomyasis (infestation with the screw worm fly) was *never* sexually transmitted, these occurrences are unusual.

Two infestations are known to be sexually transmitted, crabs and scabies. Neither *has* to be passed on this way, indeed there are outbreaks of scabies in families, nursing homes, nunneries and hospital wards, but it is rare for crabs to be caught other than during sex.

## Case history

Mr M-M, an African businessman, arrived in clinic complaining of painful lumps on his penis for three days. His last sexual contact had been with a female colleague in Kenya two weeks previously when a condom had been used throughout intercourse. He had spent the following ten days with his parents at their farm outside Nairobi and had returned to England three days ago. His immaculate linen suit was, as fashion dictates, unpressed. He had never had any sexually transmitted infection in the past although, as a sexually active single man, he attended the clinic every year or so for a general check-up including an HIV test.

He was seen by a very experienced female doctor who spent half her time working in the GUM clinic and half at the nearby A&E department. Having listened to his story, she asked him to remove his trousers and underwear and proceeded to examine his genitalia. There was no urethral discharge but there were three spots on the shaft of the penis, rather like boils, which were oozing a tiny bit of blood-stained fluid. He also had some tender inguinal lymph glands on the left side.

The first thing we knew of this story was an ear-splitting scream (the doctor, not the patient) coming from the examination room. She had applied a little pressure to one of the spots, to obtain some fluid for the laboratory, when a wriggling maggot, 2 cm in length, emerged from the boil. The other two 'spots' released their tumbu fly larvae after some Vaseline™ had been applied to them.

Myasis is the infestation of a living animal by the larva of a fly, in this case *Cordylobia anthropophaga*. The tumbu fly lays its eggs on drying clothes on a clothesline and they will be destroyed by ironing. Unfortunately, Mr M-M's mother had ironed neither his suit nor his underpants.

## The crab louse (*Phthirus pubis*)

Pubic lice, the 'butterflies of love', like their cousins, head and body lice, are small insects which have adapted to a parasitic lifestyle. Crab lice are sexually transmitted. Very rarely, there is a convincing story of having slept in a soiled bed and catching them that way. Very rarely. The reason for their virtually exclusive sexual mode of transmission is a combination of an inability to live for long away from their human hosts, coupled with great sloth. Crabs move at a snail's pace – unlike their larger namesakes, they do not scuttle.

The incubation period, the time between catching and noticing, is usually between two and four weeks and results from the louse's lifestyle. When there is close contact between infectable hairs, usually pubic, the adult louse transfers across and the female will soon begin to lay eggs, 'nits', which are cemented to other pubic hairs. These hatch and, in their turn, become adults and start to reproduce. It is not until this cycle has been repeated several times that the sheer number of lice makes their presence known.

The lice are tiny, not much more than a millimetre in length, flat and never seem to move when you watch them. The nits are much smaller, and are laid at the base of a hair. By the time they are ready to hatch, the hair will have grown a little and taken them away from the skin surface.

Pubic lice are different from body or head lice and, in general, are found only in pubic hair and the hair around the anus. Rarely they may infect the eyelashes or eyebrows and, in particularly hairy people, may infest body hair as well. They are virtually never found in head hair.

The reason crab lice stick almost exclusively to the anogenital region is, appropriately, a sexual one. Pubic hairs are further apart than hairs elsewhere on the body particularly when compared to hairs on the head. For successful coitus to take place, the male and female lice each grab two adjacent hairs with two pairs of rear legs, front to front. This juxtaposition is impossible if the hairs are too close together, as on the scalp.

## What will I notice and how is it diagnosed?

The crab louse infestation causes itching, largely in the pubic area. It may take a day or two of itching before the horrible realization arises that there are little beasts crawling about and then it is a mad dash to the clinic. Once the possibility has arisen, simple inspection suffices to confirm the diagnosis. It is possible to examine a louse using a microscope with a weak lens but this is usually unnecessary.

There are usually more female lice than males on an infested person and the males are relatively promiscuous. The female lays up to fifty eggs at perhaps three per day. She grabs a hair and deposits some 'cement' which is extruded just before she lays the egg. This glue is very powerful and will not be removed by hot water, soaps or detergents.

In only about a quarter of cases have the patients actually seen the lice. The itching may not be due to the insects moving over the skin but to an allergic reaction set up to the lice or their faeces. There may be a rash due to scratching and sometimes faint bluish spots develop at the site of louse bites. These may last for a few days.

At about two millimetres across, the crab louse is often difficult to see and because it is so flat it can easily be mistaken for a small mole on the skin. Once detached, their legs are seen to move. They are naturally a brown colour but, after feeding on blood, they may take on a reddish tinge.

When the lice infest the eyelashes or eyebrows, there may be a marked blepharitis, inflammation around the eye, which can be difficult to diagnose and is resistant to treatment until the correct diagnosis is made. Careful examination will reveal the tell-tale nits attached to the hairs.

## What is the treatment?

Virtue's *Household Physician* of 1924 suggests: 'the main object in the treatment of these filthy diseases is the destruction of the parasite . . . strict cleanliness of the person is a *sine qua non* . . . the remedies usually employed are the mercurials, sulphur, carbolic acid, tobacco, etc.' In reality, none of these remedies is effective, and cleanliness, while indeed close to godliness, does not lead to louselessness.

Treatment consists of applying one of the liquids or creams that kill the louse to the affected hairy parts. In the old days DDT gave a reliable cure and benzyl benzoate or gamma-benzene hexachloride were certainly more effective than carbolic acid or tobacco. More modern agents include permethrin and malathion, which will be familiar to gardeners as a treatment for greenfly on roses. These products kill both the adult lice and their eggs but will not remove the nits from the hairs. If these must go then shaving, carefully, or a close friend with a fine-toothed comb will do the trick. The products mentioned above can be harmful if in contact with the eyes – if you think your eyebrows or eyelashes are infested it is best to go to your GP or a GUM clinic. Treated patients tend to return to clinic a week or so later demanding further treatment because the nits, although dead, remain attached to the hairs.

There are no complications associated with crabs – they do not act, like mosquitoes, as carriers of disease – but as the lice are sexually acquired, it is sensible to attend a GUM clinic for screening. Two out of five people with crabs will have another sexually transmitted disease.

## Scabies (*Sarcoptes scabeii*)

Scabies, the 'Royal itch', is in the list of STIs under slightly false pretences. While it *can* be sexually transmitted, it is certainly passed on much more frequently in non-sexual circumstances. The itch is not painful and James

I (hence the 'Royal') claimed that the itch was fit only for kings, so exquisite was the enjoyment of scratching.

## What causes it?

The female of *Sarcoptes scabei*, var *hominis*, to give the mite of scabies its full Latin name, is some four millimetres in length, twice the size of the male. It has eight legs and is a member of the class *Arachnida*, which includes spiders and scorpions. Different mammalian species have their own varieties of scabetic mite

## Who gets scabies?

Like crabs, close physical contact is needed for transmission but this does not have to be between the genitals. Schoolchildren pass it on holding hands, nurses catch it moving patients on a ward and it can infest whole families with ease. The mite that causes scabies is much smaller than the crab louse and has a different lifestyle. Once contact is made with a new host, the mite burrows through the skin where it resides, laying eggs. These hatch, emerge on the surface of the skin, copulate and the females burrow again to repeat the cycle.

Because the scabies mite prefers loose skin, it has particular sites of preference on the body. The finger webs, wrists, breasts and buttocks are favourites, but so are the genitals. The skin of the penis and foreskin suit the mite particularly well and this may explain scabies' place in a list of STIs.

## What are the signs and symptoms?

The main symptom is itching, serious itching, which is not confined to the genital area. Indeed, in most cases, the itch will be elsewhere as long as it is below the head and neck. The cause of the itch is not the mite moving or burrowing but a hypersensitivity reaction, an allergy, to the mite and its excrement. This may take weeks rather than days, by which time, just as with crabs, cycles of reproduction have taken place and the mite may have spread over much of the body.

The itching is so intense it is almost impossible not to scratch. Scratching leads to removal of the outermost layer of the skin, which may lead to secondary bacterial infection and nasty, sometimes weeping, swollen sores. If these are on the penis it is not unnatural to assume some awful venereal disease.

## How is the diagnosis made?

The history and distribution of the itch, and even the sight of the mites' burrows, make a clinical diagnosis easy in most cases, particularly if partners or family members are similarly affected. In a GUM clinic, the burrow can be 'de-roofed', an adult mite and/or its eggs can be hooked out and it can be seen clearly using a microscope.

## What is the treatment?

The same products used for crab lice work equally well with scabies. Permethrin, malathion or similar compounds are effective and must be applied to the whole body surface for twelve hours. Because the itch is due to an allergy, killing the mites and their eggs does not get rid of the itch, which may take several days to disappear.

No serious complications occur but the skin lesions may become infected with bacteria, secondary to the scratching that occurs, and may need antibiotic treatment.

## Molluscum contagiosum (MC)

Molluscum contagiosum is a viral skin condition that, like scabies, sits somewhat uncomfortably in a list of sexually transmitted infections. The virus belongs to a group known as the pox viruses. In spite of this seemingly happy coincidence, it is by no means always sexually transmitted although like scabies it *can* be passed on that way and is thought more likely to be so when the spots are on or near the genitals. However, more often than not, MC has been passed on innocently by casual contact of a non-sexual fashion. Once the infection is present, it may be spread by scratching; a problem for those who shave their pubic hair, which makes it difficult to eradicate.

Many more people suffer from MC than are reported from GUM clinics as a majority are seen by general practitioners or dermatologists.

## What are the signs and symptoms?

There is a wide incubation period from two weeks to six months. Molluscum contagiosum has a characteristic appearance. The spots are pink, raised and have a 'pearly' sheen on the tops. They also have a little dip on the surface (i.e. they are umbilicated, like the navel). It is possible to confirm the diagnosis by using an electron microscope to identify the virus but in 99.9 per cent of cases the characteristic appearance of the spots is enough.

They vary in size from two to five millimetres (rarely even a centimetre across) and as many as 30 or 40 may be present at one time.

The collections of small raised spots may itch a little but, more usually, it is simply their unexpected presence and spreading that is noticed. It appears that persons with HIV infection are more likely to suffer bad outbreaks of MC on the face.

## What is the treatment?

The spots can be frozen using liquid nitrogen spray in the same manner as wart treatment. An alternative is to pierce the centres of the spots (which contain a white, cheesy material) with a sharpened orange stick dipped in liquid phenol.

Freezing or 'phenolizing' may sometimes leave a small scar or small area of depigmentation which may be more noticeable in dark skin.

This is a benign condition that is likely to improve even without any treatment after some months.

## Gay bowel syndrome

Sexually transmitted diarrhoea was first reported from the West Coast of America in the mid-1970s and given the catchy but inaccurate epithet of 'gay bowel syndrome'. Inaccurate because it is a sexual behaviour rather than a sexual orientation that determines the likelihood of acquiring this collection of infections. Anilingus is not restricted to homosexual men any more than is receptive rectal intercourse.

There are three principal bacterial infections (there could be others but these are the ones commonly identified), salmonellosis, shigellosis and campylobacter infection, and one viral, hepatitis A, which is dealt with below. Each of these diseases is passed on by the so-called 'faeco-oral' route. Under normal circumstances this describes food poisoning passed on to unfortunate diners by chefs, kitchen workers and other food handlers as a result of poor hygiene – not washing their hands after use of the toilet. Direct contact of tongue to anus 'cuts out the middle man' and serves as a particularly efficient and direct way of passing on infection.

There are also three protozoal diseases that may be passed on by this route. Giardiasis (caused by *Giardia lamblia*) is found more often in gay than straight men although the infection is often symptomless. Amoebic dysentery (*Entamoeba hystolitica)* and cryptosporidiosis (*Cryptosporidium parvum*) make up the trio but sexual transmission is not as certain for these two.

Finally, a nematode, *Enterobius vermicularis*, also known as the thread-worm or pinworm, can be efficiently passed on during sexual activity. We are used to seeing this condition in young children with itchy bottoms but it is just as happy infesting an adult as a child.

## Cytomegalovirus (CMV)

Properly known as human cytomegalovirus (HCMV), CMV is, like herpes simplex, herpes zoster and chicken pox, a member of the herpes family of viruses and causes few problems in those with an intact immune system. By adulthood nearly 100 per cent of those in less developed countries and 50 per cent of humans worldwide will be infected.

## How is it caught?

If CMV is not acquired from breast milk, then contact with other children in playgroups will produce the infection. In adulthood sexual transmission is the most common mode. Blood transfusion or organ transplant are other efficient ways of transmitting this virus.

## What does CMV do?

Well, in most cases, absolutely nothing. Rather like that of HSV, a primary CMV infection in childhood may produce no symptoms at all. In some it produces an illness very similar to glandular fever, which is caused by yet another herpes virus, Ebstein-Barr. In developed countries where disease prevalence is low, primary infection can occur in older adults, a difficult diagnosis to think of.

CMV's importance arises in those whose immune system is less than perfect. Recipients of kidney, liver or other solid organs have their immunity deliberately reduced so that the transplant is not rejected, as do those who receive bone marrow. Those with HIV infection are similarly susceptible to CMV, which will often have been present for some time anyway but needed the immunosuppression of AIDS to allow it to cause illness.

Before the advent of treatment (see Chapter 12 on HAART) 25 per cent of people living with AIDS developed CMV in the retina which leads inexorably to blindness. Involvement of the nervous system and gastroin-testinal tract are also likely.

Blood tests are available for diagnosis and, if in doubt, biopsy specimens show typical appearances. There are several antiviral drugs which are effective in CMV infection including ganciclovir and foscarnet but nowadays good treatment of the HIV infection is the best way to control CMV.

# Hepatitis A, B and C

Hepatitis simply means an '-itis', or inflammation, of the liver. This may be due to many causes, some infectious, some chemical, some unexplained. It may seem strange to have a section on hepatitis among a host of sexually related conditions but there are two viral forms, hepatitis A and B, that may be sexually transmitted under certain circumstances. A third viral form, hepatitis C, is mentioned briefly as a small number of those attending GUM clinics are infected with it, or think that they may be and there is continuing debate as to the role of sex in its transmission.

# Who gets viral hepatitis?

Hepatitis A is the classical 'food poisoning' form of hepatitis and most cases are caught by people who have eaten or drunk something that has been prepared under unhygienic conditions by somebody who is themselves acutely infected with the virus. So, not surprisingly, there can be outbreaks centred on a kitchen in a busy restaurant or spread within families. Rather than using food as a 'taxi' to take the virus from one person to another, transmission can occur directly by oral sex if the mouth or tongue comes into close proximity with the anus. This form of sexual transmission occurs in both sexes and in those of either sexual orientation but is most common in homosexual men.

Hepatitis B is not spread so readily but can be highly infectious given the right circumstances – some say that it is one thousand times more infectious than HIV. There are three main ways by which hepatitis B is spread. The first is by contamination with infected blood, or blood products such as factor VIII for haemophiliacs. All blood and blood products are routinely tested for hepatitis B and the risk in the UK of infection by this means is effectively zero. Injecting drug users (IDUs) who share needles or syringes are at particular risk of hepatitis B (and HepC) because of blood contamination.

The second mode of transmission occurs in parts of the world where hepatitis B is 'endemic', that is to say widespread and ever present, such as Africa, South-East Asia, the Mediterranean, Eastern Europe and Central and South America. In these endemic areas the virus is spread by vertical (mother to unborn baby) and horizontal (between persons, including sexually) spread.

The last way that hepatitis B spreads is sexually, most efficiently by anal intercourse. This seems a particularly efficient method of transmission perhaps because of the small tears and abrasions that can occur. Homosexual men are thus especially at risk.

Hepatitis C is, like hepatitis B, passed on by blood products and can be passed on sexually by gay men. Mother-to-infant transmission occurs occasionally when the mother is HIV-positive.

## What are the signs and symptoms?

The incubation period of hepatitis A is two to six and a half weeks and most infected people have minor or no symptoms giving no clue as to the diagnosis. Others may develop a flu-like illness which may progress to frank yellow jaundice with pale motions and dark urine. The right upper side of the abdomen may be sore, that is where the liver is found, and this stage may last for two weeks or longer. A very small number develop a life-threatening liver failure.

Hepatitis B, like A, may produce no symptoms. For those who do become unwell, the illness may take up to five or six months to show itself although most cases show themselves earlier. The signs and symptoms, for those who develop them, are like those of hepatitis A.

Hepatitis C only rarely produces symptoms when infection occurs and in a majority there will be no indication that infection has taken place.

## Are there any complications of the condition?

Hepatitis A is a self-limiting disease which is followed by return to full health and immunity from further attacks.

Hepatitis B is like hepatitis A in most cases with full health and immunity following infection. However, in a number of cases the virus is not eliminated from the body and a 'carrier' state ensues. Such a state is variably infectious (see below) and may lead, at its worst, to liver damage culminating in cirrhosis of the liver

Up to 85 per cent of those infected with hepatitis C become chronic carriers of the virus (and therefore potentially infectious to others). It used to be thought that 25 per cent of these chronic carriers of hepatitis C would go on to permanent liver damage after 20 years or so but it now appears that this figure is probably too high and the outlook is not so grim.

# How is it diagnosed?

The mainstay of diagnosis for all three forms of hepatitis is blood testing that looks for antibodies against each virus, or identification of particular parts of a virus (such as 'e' or 's' antigen). A combination of tests can determine whether infection is current, in the past, chronic, or absent and whether vaccination, in the case of hepatitis A and hepatitis B, is indicated.

Dealing with hepatitis A is straightforward. Once infected, a person will never catch hepatitis A again, so the presence of antibodies in the blood test betokens immunity, whether they result from natural infection or from vaccination. Vaccination consists of two intramuscular injections at an interval of six months.

The next two paragraphs are intensely boring unless you have a personal interest in hepatitis B and other readers are well advised to skip them.

Hepatitis B is more complicated then hepatitis A and the blood tests are poorly understood by many doctors and nurses, let alone patients. If somebody has never been infected with hepatitis B and never been vaccinated, there are no antibodies in the blood. Simple. When an infection has occurred in the past (and remember, this may have caused no symptoms at the time), there will be antibodies to the 'core' of the virus, hepatitis B core *antibody*, or *hepatitis B cAb*, for short. If the patient fully recovered, there will also be another test showing antibodies to hepatitis B *surface* antigen, *hepatitis B sAb*. All other tests will be negative.

If, however, some viral infection persists, it will be possible to detect part of the virus itself, the surface *antigen*, in shorthand, *hepatitis B sAg*. If surface antigen is detected this means that there is still active virus present in the body and the person in question is a chronic carrier and infectious but not greatly so. There is a further blood test which looks for antibodies to the 'e' antigen, *hepatitis B eAb*, which will also be positive in the persons of 'low infectivity'. Detection, however, of the 'e' *antigen*, *hepatitis B eAg*, means very high infectivity, enough to ban a surgeon from ever operating again, for example.

Hepatitis C is diagnosed using a highly sensitive antibody test with confirmation by a test that identifies hepatitis C RNA.

# Is there any treatment?

Prevention is better than cure. Vaccination is recommended for those at particular risk and male homosexuals or heterosexual partners of chronic hepatitis B carriers, are offered this treatment in GUM clinics. The clinics will *not*, however, vaccinate low-risk persons who simply wish to protect themselves against food poisoning abroad. There are moves afoot to institute universal hepatitis B vaccination in the UK because of increasing numbers of cases but there is little evidence of ongoing transmission within low-risk groups.

Those with evidence of carriage of hepatitis B or C will have tests of how well their liver is functioning and if there is evidence of deterioration, various antiviral agents can be used. Interferon-alpha gives improvement in up to 40 per cent of cases of hepatitis B with complete cure in 10 per cent. Some reverse-transcriptase inhibitors (see Chapter 12) including lamivudine have shown some good effect. In hepatitis C infection, combining interferon with ribavirin has had some striking successes but only in a minority of cases.

## Resources

www.bashh.org/guidelines.htm

# 11 The story of HIV and AIDS

## What are HIV infection and AIDS, and who catches them?

To understand today's global problem with HIV infection, and to see what might happen and where the epidemic might go next, we can learn much from the way in which the infection has spread both in geographical terms and between and among different sections of the human community. Unhappy as it makes the advocates of the 'everybody's at equal risk' interpretation, some people and some behaviours carry with them a measurably increased chance of both acquiring and transmitting HIV infection.

A seemingly innocuous little article published in 1981 in a US public health journal, *Morbidity and Mortality Weekly Report* (*MMWR*), which first brought the condition caused by the human immunodeficiency virus (HIV) to the attention of the medical profession. '*Pneumocystis* pneumonia – Los Angeles' was the dry title and it centred on a neat piece of detective work by medical epidemiologists, those who count and measure disease trends. Pentamidine is an intravenous drug used to treat a severe lung infection, *Pneumocystis carinii* pneumonia (PCP), which occurs in some patients following kidney transplantation. Because PCP was a rare event, pentamidine had to be obtained specially from a central supply and our sleuths noticed that more than was expected was being ordered in Los Angeles.

Their inquiries revealed that the five treated cases in Los Angeles were not transplant patients but homosexual men. It was known that transplant patients developed PCP because their immune system had been weakened with drugs (deliberately) to reduce the chances of rejection of their new kidney. None of the men was taking such medication, so it looked as if their immune system was being weakened in some other way. Soon after, a strange tumour of blood-forming tissue, Kaposi's sarcoma, was detected in increasing numbers, again in homosexual men.

Within the year a multitude of new cases had been reported from San Francisco and New York to add to the increasing number in Los Angeles. A few sporadic cases had occurred in the UK by the end of 1982 but the large majority were in the USA, most of them in homosexual men. Most of them, but not all.

## The four 'H's

AIDS was seen to be affecting four main groups of people: homosexuals, heroin addicts, haemophiliacs and Haitians. The puzzling thing was not that they all began with 'H' but that Haitians, in the main heterosexual, constituted a risk group. The risk for haemophiliacs and injecting drug users (IDUs) could be explained if there was an infectious agent, probably a virus, in blood and blood products. IDUs shared needles and syringes, and haemophiliacs controlled their bleeding tendency by injecting themselves with factor VIII which had come from pooled donated blood. But Haitians?

The Haitian cases were reported from New York and Miami, the two conurbations with the largest number of Haitian immigrants. The disease was most common in those who had been only a short time in the USA – the average time was just over two years – and whose mean age was thirty, 3–6 years younger than infected homosexuals and haemophiliacs. Thirty per cent were women. This lent support for heterosexual activity as a mode of transmission at a time when sections of the media were at pains to label the new disease 'gay compromise syndrome'.

One explanation was that Haiti acted as a staging post in the passage of HIV from Africa to the USA. When the Belgian Congo became independent, Zaire, the new nation, having freed itself largely of European influence, was in need of teachers, civil servants, middle management, etc., who would be able to speak French. Francophone Haiti was a convenient source and there was a lot of interchange and much travel between the two countries. It looked as though Zaire and the Central African Republic were close to the epicentre of HIV-1 spread. Like an earthquake whose ripples can be traced back to the centre of the shock, AIDS cases during the early 1980s appeared to be spreading from that geographical area.

While most of the Haitians were heterosexual, a few were not and Haiti was a popular holiday resort for homosexual New Yorkers. It is possible that young, poor, Haitian men may have been the unwitting conduit for the infection between Africa and America, via this Caribbean island. Whatever the connection, once in the USA, the spread was rapid with a well-documented route of HIV transmission from an infected New York gay man to several contacts on the West Coast.

# Where did HIV come from?

HIV infection originated in the continent of Africa. Let it be said early that HIV infection is neither a result of some grim CIA plan to take over the world (and, while we are debunking crack-pot theories, HIV *is* the virus that causes AIDS), nor was it spread through Africa by polio immunizations in the 1980s. Conspiracy theorists have produced these and other explanations for the global pandemic but the truth is simpler, if less attractive to those with a political rather than a scientific agenda.

The first infection of a man or woman with HIV must have occurred decades before the US cases were recognized in 1981. HIV is very similar to SIV, simian immunodeficiency virus, which is known to infect monkeys in parts of Africa. Because each virus evolves at a particular rate, it is possible to use mathematical backtracking to calculate how long it would have taken for SIV to change to HIV. This seems to have happened within the sixty years before AIDS first emerged in the USA. There is more than one SIV so, for example, the virus that affects the green monkey is unable to infect humans, whereas that transmitted by the sooty mangabey can. This monkey's SIV is quite similar to HIV-2, a variant discovered in 1986 in West Africa. On the other hand, HIV-1 seems to be derived from an SIV found in chimpanzees.

The ability of some viruses to evolve and change over time, *viz.* SIV to HIV, is one of the reasons that it has been so difficult to make an effective vaccine to HIV. It is possible to manufacture antibodies to HIV that ought to work but, by the time enough are made, the goalposts have been moved and HIV is no longer the same target. This ability to evolve also explains the problems faced with resistance to antiviral drugs which can develop amazingly quickly if the wrong combinations or levels of drugs are given.

# Why did it spread so fast?

The chances of transmitting HIV vary depending on certain circumstances, some behavioural, others to do with the amount of virus in the body, the viral load. Injecting HIV directly into the bloodstream as happens with factor VIII or a contaminated syringe, is the most efficient. Rectal intercourse is riskier than vaginal intercourse which is riskier than oral sex. Perhaps the most important variable, however, is the amount of virus present. After infection there is a period of some weeks, perhaps two to six, during which time antibodies develop in the blood. This seroconversion period coincides with just about the largest number of viruses in the body that occur at any stage of the illness. The more viruses there are, the more likely is the infection to be passed on.

If HIV is introduced to a group of people who are sharing risk at a high rate, then most will be seroconverting with a high viral load during the risk-sharing and transmission will be that more efficient. Two examples: In the late 1970s and early 1980s, there existed in California a notorious 'bath-house' scene for gay men. Alcohol and recreational drugs abounded, the lighting was low and the clothing was light, if at all, and casual couplings were the order of the day and night. I was told by some of my British patients who had been to San Francisco around that time that three partners per night was not unusual, every night. Hundreds of sexual contacts a year. Introduce HIV into that scene and it will spread rapidly. The other example was the increase among IDUs in Edinburgh in the early 1980s where the prevalence of HIV infection rose from 1.5 per cent in 1983 to 55 per cent in 1985.

So, those who are seroconverting are more likely to pass on HIV because more virus is present in their bodies during that time. Later on in HIV infection, if it has not been controlled by antiretroviral drugs, the viral load and infectiousness begin to rise again. When other infections occur, like tuberculosis or meningitis, viral load also begins to increase. This also applies to other sexually transmitted diseases which, when active, are accompanied by the excretion of more virus and make the person more infectious.

## What does HIV do?

Human immunodeficiency virus is a retrovirus and, like all viruses, depends for its energy on infecting a living cell. HIV happens to use a specialized technique, once inside the cell, to reproduce itself. The genetic code of cells is carried as DNA (deoxyribonucleic acid), Watson and Crick's famous double helix. HIV, however, is made up of RNA, a different sort of nucleic acid, so it needs somehow to convert this to DNA in order to incorporate itself into the cell's chromosome. Reverse transcriptase is an enzyme that does just that. Enzymes are facilitators that enable biological changes to take place in animals and plants, and usually end in '-ase'. Thus lipase helps digest lipid fats, and amylase breaks down starch. Using reverse transcriptase, the virus becomes part of the host cell's DNA where it can remain latent until called upon to reproduce itself.

HIV has an affinity for certain sorts of cells, those with CD4 receptors. These include a particular white cell, the T-cell, which is crucial in the efficient running of the body's immune system. It is the infection and subsequent death of these T-cells that is mainly responsible for the immunodeficiency which HIV causes. CD4 lymphocytes are the prime target for HIV but macrophages, another sort of white cell, Langerhans cells, found in mucous membranes and the foreskin, and some cells, the microgliae, found in the brain are also susceptible to infection. The presence of CD4 receptors in cells in the foreskin has lent credence to the observation that HIV transmission seems less common in Africa in circumcised men than in uncircumcised. This holds true even when other risk factors and religion have been taken into account.

No matter what cell is infected by HIV, after a variable time it will be forced to produce more virus in the process of which it will die.

## Who catches HIV infection?

The simple answer, and that loved by the propagandists of the 1980s, is that *anyone* can. It is certainly true that anybody *can*, but not everybody does. Further, different people seem at different risk in different parts of the world. I deal with the various risk groups and risk activities in the order in which they emerged and became apparent.

The first epidemic to be described in detail was that in gay men in the USA. As noted above, they still remain the largest group to suffer from HIV/AIDS in that part of the world. Likewise, the first cases in the UK and in Europe were found in gay men. Unprotected anal intercourse, riskier for the receiver than for the inserter, is a more efficient way of passing on HIV than vaginal sex.

In the USA, injecting drug users, particularly those who share equipment, currently come a close second in numbers to men who have sex with men. The expected increase in IDUs with HIV in Western Europe has not happened but this risk group predominates in Eastern Europe and in parts of the Far East.

The risk of HIV infection in haemophiliacs was high in the days before an antibody test enabled blood to be tested for HIV. New infections in this group, like those from blood transfusions (never a major contributor to the epidemic), are virtually unheard of today. As a measure of how uninfectious HIV is (compared to, say, hepatitis B), the number of cases of 'needlestick' infection, passed on to nurses or surgeons by pricking or cutting themselves with a needle or scalpel contaminated with blood from an infected person, has been very small worldwide.

Bisexual men were initially seen along with IDUs as a 'bridge' from high risk groups into the general population, but have not actually been a numerically important group other than in Central and South American countries where the so-called 'macho' culture, common to that part of the Americas, does not allow open homosexuality. There, gay men may feel obliged to marry in order to mask their preferred sexual orientation. Similar pressures exist in the Caribbean.

Lastly, and most significantly, heterosexuals. Worldwide, cases due to heterosexual transmission vastly outnumber those in all the other categories put together. Sub-Saharan Africa has the largest number of sufferers of HIV/AIDS and, in that region, the epidemic is almost exclusively heterosexually driven. Vertical transmission of HIV, from mother to unborn child (or, rarely, as a result of breast-feeding), is seen in those parts of the world where heterosexual transmission is common. Nowadays such vertical transmission can be largely prevented using antiretroviral drugs, if and when these drugs are made available.

So, we see risk activities associated with risk groups but closer analysis shows an uneven spread of infection even within the different groupings. Do all heroin addicts have an equal risk of infection? Are all gay men as likely to catch HIV? Is the probability of infection the same for all heterosexuals in Africa or, for that matter, in Seattle, in Trinidad or in the UK? The answer to all these questions is 'No'. Throughout the world there are racial and ethnic differences in rates of infection. These are due to combinations of local circumstances, behavioural differences and simple factors such as the provision and uptake of health care rather than any supposed genetic susceptibilities.

Taking the whole of the USA in 1999, an African-American was 6.6 times more likely to be infected than a White American, the ratio varying between 2.9 times more likely in California to 16 times in Pennsylvania. In the UK it took some time for this politically incorrect, differential risk to be accepted with the result that neither heterosexual positives (predominantly Black) nor homosexual men (predominantly White) received the targeted health care or health advice that should have been theirs of right, until well into the 1990s.

## The epidemic in the USA

The first report of PCP in five gay men was published in the *MMWR* in 1981. By June 1982, over 400 further cases of AIDS had been found. Remembering that in those days it took around ten years to develop AIDS after initial HIV infection and that HIV cases would outnumber AIDS ones by at least five to one, this gives an idea of just how far the epidemic had progressed and that it must already have been around for several years in the USA. The Centers for Disease Control (CDC) in Atlanta are responsible for the collection of HIV and AIDS figures (as well as epidemiological data on other infections and public health matters). Members of staff at the CDC were the detectives who had followed up the original five Los Angeles cases.

By 1984 some differences were emerging between the reported cases in the USA and the UK. In the USA 17 per cent of AIDS cases were in IDUs and 3 per cent, all Haitians, were associated with Africa and the Caribbean, compared with one IDU only in the UK but 6 per cent associated with Africa. In Europe the number of cases associated with Africa made up an even greater proportion. Much vital research was taking place in the USA including the invention of a blood test, at last, that identified antibodies to HIV in blood. This advance had not been possible until the virus responsible for AIDS was identified in the laboratory.

The 'possible' virus had been named HTLV-III by an American expert in retroviruses, Robert Gallo. He published details of this virus in 1983, to worldwide scientific acclaim, at much the same time as a French virologist, Luc Montagnier, whose laboratory was at the Institut Pasteur in Paris. A public scandal ensued when it transpired that the virus 'discovered' by Gallo was identical to one that Montagnier had previously sent him, as a courtesy. The other name for HIV at that time was LAV, lymphadenopathy associated virus, which reflected the fact that many people's glands were enlarged during infection. LAV and HTLV-III were renamed HIV in 1986.

In the 1980s San Francisco was home to a large number of HIV-infected homosexual men and this put considerable pressure on the available health resources. There developed a widespread desire to contribute and help and a system of care for HIV-infected individuals was developed that served as a model, in later years, for a better level of service provision in the USA and abroad. While units in the UK were putting their resources into the provision of inpatient care with dedicated AIDS wards springing up in all the best hospitals, the San Francisco General Hospital (SFGH) was concentrating on keeping infected individuals out. The first topic for discussion when a patient was admitted to SFGH's Ward 5 was when they could be discharged. There was also a keen desire to involve patients in their own care, to allow them to be part of any decision-making process.

In the UK at the time, many physicians were appalled at the suggestion that a patient should be told about, let alone asked for permission for, an HIV test. 'Damn it, we don't discuss haemoglobin tests or cancer investigations...' was a typical reaction. Probably the only good thing to have come out of the HIV epidemic was a sea change, prompted by the positive gay community, in the degree of patient involvement, not just those with HIV, in decisions about their own health.

The epidemic in America moved rapidly from a predominantly male homosexual one to the current situation of high numbers of drug-related cases and a significant proportion of heterosexually acquired infections. As in the UK, it is ethnic minorities, in this case African-American and Hispanic, who are disproportionately involved as are an increasing number of women. Recent research from New York City showed that women were twice as likely to be infected by a husband or steady boyfriend as by casual sex partners. For all that, the majority of persons who are alive and HIV-infected in the USA are gay men.

It is worth repeating that race and ethnicity are not in themselves risk factors for HIV. Poverty and socioeconomic deprivation are strongly related to risk. Up-to-date figures and breakdowns of risk groups can be found at the UNAIDS website.

## The epidemic in the UK

The Communicable Disease Surveillance Centre (CDSC) is the UK equivalent of the Centers for Disease Control in the USA and, like the CDC, has been responsible for collecting HIV/AIDS figures since the start of the epidemic. As in America the British epidemic started with homosexual men but, by contrast, in the UK it was known where the infection had come from – the USA. British gay men had been envious of the uncluttered, free approach to sex on the West Coast and, by mid-1983, seven of the first twelve homosexual AIDS cases had had sex with men in the USA. The only haemophiliac case had used factor VIII from America. By February 1985, there were 132 AIDS cases of which 117 were in gay men, three were haemophiliac and six were connected with Africa in some way.

Although it lagged behind, the UK epidemic mirrored that of the USA with a predominantly male homosexual contribution and an increasing number of IDU-related cases. It was accepted, after a struggle, that supplying clean needles and syringes to IDUs was an obvious way of reducing person to person transmission and needle exchange facilities became increasingly available. Moralists complained that by doing so, society was not only condoning misuse of drugs but encouraging it. Realists just got on with reducing infection rates.

By the end of 1986, a total of 3877 HIV-positives had been reported, including 1964 gay men, 217 IDUs, 930 haemophiliacs and 48 heterosexuals.

This increasing number of infected heterosexuals was to become the focus of much attention and provide authority to public health campaigns for safer sex in the general population.

A subtle yet important change occurred in the way in which the number of cases was reported, just prior to a massive country-wide anti-AIDS publicity campaign. Until the end of 1986, most of the heterosexuals in the CDSC's monthly HIV reports were identified by a footnote that said '... associated with sub-Saharan Africa'. This footnote was missing from tables published in November 1986 and heterosexual AIDS cases were simply subdivided into 'presumed infected abroad' and 'presumed infected UK'. The December HIV tables simply had a category for 'heterosexuals', with no sub-division.

This change in reporting categories happened one month before a nationwide leaflet drop, in January 1987, to every household in the UK, part of the 'Don't die of ignorance' campaign. Much was made of the increasing number of heterosexual cases and it was possible to assume, as many people did, egged on by the media, that heterosexual cases *reported* were the same as heterosexual cases *transmitted* within the UK. Further, there was a tacit assumption that those who had caught HIV in sub-Saharan Africa were UK nationals who had travelled there, rather than citizens of African countries.

This loss of the 'African connection' in the reported figures lasted until the early 1990s, with two important consequences. It enabled the myth of an ever-increasing epidemic of heterosexual HIV transmission in the UK to be convincingly promulgated and it denied health targeting to a particularly vulnerable section of the community. Although the figures have been quite transparent since the mid-1990s, each year the media still talk of the massive HIV epidemic as if transmission is occurring predominantly in the UK.

What then is the truth? As part of the Health Protection Agency (HPA) the figures are readily available at the CDSC's website and are to be found in the 'unpublished quarterly tables' which are updated every three months. The majority of heterosexuals in the UK with HIV/AIDS acquired their infection in sub-Saharan Africa and, of the new cases reported each year (currently running at about 4000) only a small minority, perhaps less than 150, were actually caught in the UK from someone themselves infected within Europe. An unknown percentage of the total will be infections passed from one person from a high-risk area to another from the same place.

So should we be complacent about heterosexual transmission of HIV in the UK? Absolutely not. We have been spared the degree of infection seen elsewhere for a variety of favourable circumstances, not least of which is the (comparatively) low level of other sexually transmitted diseases found in the UK. The provision of a network of clinics throughout the country, free at the point of access, has kept in check what is probably the single most important accelerator of an HIV epidemic.

What of the other risk categories? Since 1989 there have been fewer than thirty new blood factor cases annually (13 reported so far for 2004, as I write) and new IDU infections have been fewer than 200 per year since 1989 (61 in 2004). Mother to infant cases, a reflection on the heterosexual epidemic, peaked at 141 cases in 2003.

Since the year 2000 there has been a slow but steady increase in HIV infection among MSM. This has attracted little notice since the figures have been overshadowed by the greater increase in the, mostly imported, heterosexual cases. There is a suggestion that some gay men are ignoring the lessons of the past and ditching safer sex practices because of the greatly improved outlook for those with HIV since the advent of multiple drug treatment HAART. A recent patient of mine, just down from university, was shocked by the sight, in a gay club, of couples openly 'bare-backing'. When the efficacy of the condom's role in preventing transmission of HIV and other STIs has been so well established, he found it extraordinary that such risks were being taken, and so openly.

## The epidemic in Africa

There is not one but several epidemics of HIV infection in Africa. Some have almost burnt themselves out while others are yet to reach their maximum effect. However, even when a country has seen a downturn in numbers of new HIV infections, it will still have to face the epidemic of AIDS cases that invariably follows. During the 1980s, when one talked of the 'African' HIV epidemic, one always added the rider '... excluding South Africa'. This was because there was little infection at the time when Central and Eastern African countries were carrying the main burden of disease. Today (2005) South Africa is the country with the highest number of HIV-positive people in the world. Likewise, in North Africa, above the Sahara desert and in the Middle East, little infection was to be found at the start of the pandemic.

As noted above, the epicentre of HIV-1 infection was thought to be in the region of the Central African Republic and Zaire (Belgian Congo). There was more rapid spread eastwards and southwards to Uganda, Kenya, Tanzania and Zambia. For many years the largest number of heterosexually-infected individuals in the UK had acquired their infection in Uganda. Today,

Zimbabwe, Botswana and South Africa are the sites of infection most likely in new cases. The epidemic in Uganda is probably over the worst, having peaked in the late 1980s.

HIV-1 spread westwards and one could measure a steadily increasing number of cases in Nigeria, Ghana and Sierra Leone. Students of history and geography will notice that, with the exception of the Central African Republic and Zaire, all countries are past British colonies. There is a similar relationship between other European countries in respect of the geographical origin of many cases, for example, Belgium and Zaire, or France and Ivory Coast.

Why the disease has grabbed such a hold in Africa has puzzled investigators over the years. A major advance in understanding came in 1988/89 with the publication of papers showing increased transmission of HIV when there was a concurrent sexually transmitted disease. One convincing study linked the presence of chancroid, a genital ulcerative disease, with a greater chance of HIV infection. Other STIs, including gonorrhoea and other ulcers like syphilis and herpes, soon followed as important co-factors in transmission. A study in Mwanza demonstrated a significant reduction in HIV transmission when a good STI service was instituted.

In the early days, much spread of infection was attributed to the truckers who travelled the main highways and paid for sexual favours along the way. The rates of infection among commercial sex workers reached 80 or 90 per cent and one could watch the march of infection through the main towns on the arterial roads, leaking into neighbouring villages and then on into rural areas. One consistent feature, not confined to the African continent, has been the subsequent infection of wives and girlfriends. There are, on average in Africa, 13 HIV-infected women for each 10 men. If the infection is looked at in those younger than 25 years, the ratio is 36 to 10. In Ghana the figure is more than 9 to 1. It is not usually useful to try to apportion blame in these circumstances but, in one recent study from Zimbabwe and South Africa, two-thirds of women reported having had only one life-time partner and four out of five had waited until 17 before having sex (just about the world average) and four out of five said they had used a condom. Yet 40 per cent were HIV positive.

Mortality is obviously very high, registered adult deaths in South Africa went up from 272 000 in 1998 to 456 700 in 2003. A recent study has shown that the average life expectancy has dropped below 40 in nine countries including Lesotho, Botswana, Zambia and Zimbabwe.

# The epidemic in Europe

Accurate figures for HIV/AIDS have been available for rather longer from Western and Central than from Eastern Europe. The early epidemic was similar to that in the USA and UK with a predominance of cases among gay men. Imported cases from Africa made up the majority of heterosexual cases although the source countries varied for the historical reasons detailed above. Injecting drug use was more of a feature of the more southern countries, France, Germany, Spain, Italy and Greece. In London in the 1980s, more IDUs diagnosed with HIV infection had been born in Italy than in Britain. Those countries that like the UK made needle-exchange facilities available, diminished transmission significantly.

The figures for Central Europe, other than Poland, have remained fairly steady since the late 1990s but the same is not true of Eastern Europe. There are alarming rates of increase in HIV in Ukraine and the Russian Federation which have paralleled their increase in cases of infectious syphilis although the HIV epidemic is driven by IDUs. One estimate suggests that between 1–2 per cent of the entire Russian population inject drugs. In early 2004, some 80 per cent of all HIV infections had been reported to be in drug injectors. Selling sex to pay for the drug habit is the petrol on the fire of the epidemic and this leads inevitably to further heterosexual transmission.

# The epidemic in Asia

There are perhaps only one-third as many people living with HIV infection in Asia compared with Africa but the potential for spread and devastation is hugely greater. Sub-Saharan Africa is home to 10 per cent of the world's population; Asia is home to 65 per cent. As with Africa, there exist many different epidemics, at different stages of their evolution. HIV has been well and long established in Thailand, Myanmar and Cambodia as well as parts of India. Vietnam, Indonesia, Nepal and some provinces in China are just beginning their expansion while others, Sri Lanka, Pakistan and Bangladesh, for example, maintain low levels of prevalence, so far.

The China epidemic has varied features. HIV became common among those in certain provinces who sold their blood to supplement their income. Elsewhere, injecting drug use and to a lesser extent commercial sex work are the driving forces. There is widespread ignorance about preventive measures – in one survey from 2003, it was found that 40 per cent of men and women were unable to name a single way in which they could protect themselves from HIV infection. Only a small minority of MSM, 3 per cent in one survey, were found to be HIV positive, all unaware of their diagnosis.

Infection among sex workers in India has been found to be 50 per cent or more in some states. The high prevalence (up to 5 per cent) in antenatal clinic attenders in Manipur is explained by many of the women being sex partners of men who inject drugs, a risk behaviour now thought to make a greater contribution than previously. The contribution of MSM to the epidemic is smaller than in the West but a high proportion also report sex with women.

In Nepal and Vietnam the epidemic is drug-driven with widespread use of unsterile injecting equipment. Efforts in Bangladesh have demonstrated significant risk reduction (in sexual practice as well as injecting) when needle-exchange programmes were introduced.

Cambodia and Thailand have both had noted success in prevention efforts, reducing not only levels of HIV but also other STIs. In both countries the HIV incidence rate is coming down as condom usage is going up. What in Thailand was a predominantly heterosexual epidemic is now fed, but in smaller numbers, by injecting drug use. Education is urgently needed elsewhere: in Pakistan, with no significant epidemic as yet, one in three lorry drivers had never heard of condoms and in East Timor, similarly untouched by HIV so far, four of ten sex workers did not recognize a condom when shown one.

Somewhat surprisingly, there has not been a significant number of cases reported in the UK that have been acquired in Asia, either by nationals of the various countries or by visitors. This is in stark contrast with African countries and may reflect the different social and geographical make-up of infected groups in, say, India, compared with a more widespread and generalized infection in sub-Saharan Africa.

## The epidemic in the Middle East and North Africa

There were probably 100 000 new HIV infections in the Middle East and North Africa in 2004. The worst-affected country is Sudan, with its civil unrest, and most new cases are found in the south. Given its proximity to Uganda, the country with one of the earliest epidemics, it is perhaps surprising that it has taken as long as it has for HIV to take hold. The prevalence of HIV is about 2 per cent, nearly half a million people, and this represents more than four in five of all infections in this whole region. One recent study from Rumbek, in the south, revealed that only one in five people had ever heard of a condom and less than 2 per cent used a condom with a casual sexual partner.

In Libya, Tunisia and Egypt, there are comparatively few infections, those mostly associated with injecting drug use. Needle-exchange programmes are urgently needed. In Morocco, heterosexual intercourse appears to be the main route of transmission although doubt has been cast on the accuracy of the figures. Elsewhere, in Algeria, Bahrain, Oman and Kuwait, injecting drug use is the major risk factor, as it is in Iran where dramatic increases in HIV cases have occurred. In part, however, this may be due to ascertainment bias, that is, more testing for HIV. Needles and syringes have recently been made available in pharmacies, an example that should be followed elsewhere in the region.

Mixing of cultures and countries is inevitable in the oil-rich states and Saudi Arabia provides an example. Most of the HIV-positive cases in Sri Lanka are in young women who have worked in domestic service in the Middle East. They are all tested for HIV before leaving their home country but many return infected. In their spare time they have struck up relationships with other immigrant labour, often construction workers imported from African countries. They catch HIV infection and in some cases pass this on to their employers who have been known to sexually abuse them.

## The epidemic in Oceania

The majority of transmissions in Australia and New Zealand are among men who have sex with men. The small number of cases in heterosexuals have, rather like the UK, occurred in those who come from, or who have had sex in, countries with high prevalence of heterosexual transmission. HIV infection acquired heterosexually or by injecting drug use, is more common among the Aboriginal peoples in Australia who also have higher than average rates of other sexually transmitted diseases.

Papua New Guinea is a different story. In spite of variable surveillance facilities, it is apparent that rapid increases in numbers are taking place and the country has the highest prevalence of HIV in the Pacific region. Antenatal prevalence was around 2 per cent in 2003 and more new infections were reported in women than men that year. The island is shared with Papua, part of Indonesia, which has itself a high prevalence of HIV in heterosexuals. Spread is largely fuelled by commercial sex workers. Other Pacific islands have not yet experienced HIV epidemics but the high rates of other STIs suggest a fertile field ripe for planting.

# The epidemic in the Caribbean

The Caribbean is an HIV/AIDS disaster erupting before our eyes; only Africa has a higher rate of infection. Over the whole region 2.3 per cent of adults are HIV-positive and AIDS is the most common cause of death among those aged between 15 and 44. Many of the countries in the region with the highest rates of HIV infection are those with popular and developed tourism industries including Jamaica, Dominican Republic, Trinidad and Tobago, the Bahamas, Barbados and Bermuda. Add to this the fact that the epidemic is largely fuelled by heterosexual transmission with the potential for spread far beyond the region's geographical confines. Bermuda and Puerto Rica are the only countries with a significant infection rate among IDUs (up to 50 per cent in each). Homosexual transmission, although undoubtedly under-reported, is not as significant a contributor as in mainland North and South America.

Haiti featured early in the unfolding story of global HIV spread and it remains the most affected area in the region. The best surveillance measure is the prevalence of HIV in pregnant women – they have to be seen to have their babies delivered, and usually before. In Haiti this antenatal prevalence has declined from 4.5 per cent to 2.8 per cent in the past eight years, a similar drop, from 3 per cent in 1995 to 2 per cent, occurring in the Dominican Republic, with whom it shares the island of Hispaniola.

As happened in sub-Saharan Africa, the rate of infection in women has overtaken that in men, with teenage girls more than twice as likely to be infected as boys in parts of the region. Jamaica is one such country and has the second highest number of cases and deaths from AIDS, after Haiti. Disturbingly, the number of AIDS reports and deaths does not appear to be diminishing, which suggests that access to, and availability of, anti-retroviral therapy is limited. By contrast, the rate of new AIDS diagnoses has halved in the Bahamas and Barbados in the past four years. Between 1998 and 2003, deaths from AIDS in Barbados decreased from 114 to 50, hospital admissions for opportunistic infections went down by 42 per cent and vertical transmission reduced by two-thirds. These encouraging figures show that results can be achieved if resources are made available and channelled appropriately.

Cuba has avoided the rapid increase in cases seen elsewhere in the region by a combination of strict quarantine rules, limiting access of people with HIV in the 1980s (since abandoned) and ready availability of health care and antiretroviral drugs. The new cases that have been seen have been mostly in homosexual men.

The HIV/AIDS epidemic in the Caribbean will impinge increasingly on those countries which have historical, colonial connections, for example, Surinam with the Netherlands, Montserrat with France, and Jamaica, particularly, with the UK.

## Resources

For world figures: **www.unaids.org**

For UK figures: **www.hpa.org.uk**

J. Erwin, D. Smith & B. Peters, eds (2003) *Ethnicity and HIV: Prevention and Cure in Europe and the USA*. London and Atlanta: International Press.

# 12 HIV and AIDS: the clinical picture

When HIV infection first surfaced on the West Coast of America in 1981, nobody quite knew what was going on or why. The editorial in the MMWR report of 5 June, 1981 included: 'The occurrence of pneumocystis (PCP) in five previously healthy individuals without a clinically apparent underlying immunodeficiency is unusual. The fact that these patients were all homosexuals suggests an association between some aspect of homosexual lifestyle or disease acquired through sexual contact...' The reference to '*some aspect of homosexual lifestyle...*' drew a red herring across the path of those trying to make sense of a clinical conundrum.

Recreational drugs and sexual stimulants were both implicated in those early days and much time was wasted looking for some connection between nitrite inhalation and PCP. By April 1983, around the time of Luc Montagnier's discovery of HIV but before its publication, there had been 1300 cases of AIDS in the USA and an infectious agent was the likeliest cause. Many of the AIDS cases had been noted to go through a prodromal phase of AIDS known as persistent generalized lymphadenopathy (PGL), lymph glands enlarging all over the body, and AIDS-related complex (ARC), with other evidence of illness but without an AIDS-defining disease.

We have the benefit today of nearly 25 years of clinical experience of HIV infection in all its manifestations and we can better manage many of the complications of the immunodeficiency. We can treat or forestall most of the previously life-threatening infections and tumours that killed early sufferers and, with the advent of highly active antiretroviral therapy (HAART), we can deliver normal uninfected babies from HIV-positive mothers and offer a normal lifespan to many people living with HIV.

People still talk of AIDS as if it were a biological rather than a man-made concept. The definition of AIDS has changed so often (in 1985, 1987, 1993 and 2000) that it is difficult to follow trends in the number of cases. When

HAART was introduced in 1997, it rapidly reduced the number of cases of AIDS (as then defined) although it had no effect on the number of new HIV infections.

In this chapter we divide the illness associated with HIV infection into *early infection*, the first few weeks when seroconversion takes place; *asymptomatic infection*, the period when the disease lies latent and an infected person appears quite healthy; *symptomatic infection*, when illnesses, not AIDS, appear but there is a measurable immunodeficiency; and, finally, *late infection* when immunosuppression and the risk of a serious infection or tumour (both AIDS-defining illnesses) is greatest.

# Early infection

## What are the symptoms of seroconversion?

Most people who contract HIV are unaware that they have been infected. Different studies suggest that up to 90 per cent of new HIV infections are associated with symptoms; however these can be nonspecific and are often only identified in retrospect.

Whether or not symptomatic, this early stage is called seroconversion or more correctly 'primary HIV infection'. It classically occurs five days to five weeks following exposure to the virus as HIV antibodies are developing and can vary in severity. Common symptoms are 'flu-like and include prolonged fever, sore throat, enlarged lymph nodes, skin rashes, tiredness, and achy joints and muscles. Ulcers on the genitals or mouth may occur as can headaches, meningitis, diarrhoea, nausea, weight loss. Less commonly, someone who is seroconverting has symptoms severe enough to warrant admission to hospital. This acute illness can last from days to months but is usually less than two weeks in duration. Patients often don't seek medical help with these nonspecific symptoms and they settle without any treatment.

## What else could be the cause of these symptoms?

As you can see from the list above, the symptoms associated with primary HIV can be very varied and non-specific. Lots of other conditions can present in a similar way, many of them viral illnesses, including 'flu or glandular fever. Primary genital herpes and early infectious syphilis are two sexually transmitted diseases that may present with similar symptoms. It must be stressed that those who have some of the symptoms described above are *not* seroconverting in almost all cases.

There has been much publicity of late in the UK about post-exposure prophylaxis (PEP) and its role following risk of possible infection. There are certain situations when there is a quantifiable risk, for example a condom accident if one of a couple is known to be HIV-positive, a needlestick injury from an HIV patient, or sexual assault. In most other cases, the grimness of the treatment quite outweighs the risk of acquiring HIV.

## Post-exposure prophylaxis (PEP)

If there *has* been a measurable risk, time is of the essence. Anti-HIV drugs should be started within 72 hours of the possible infection to try to minimize the risk of seroconverting. This treatment will have to be continued for a month. PEP can be prescribed at A&E or at a specialist GUM clinic. So far, so good. However, there is a lack of reliable scientific evidence to support definitive guidelines on PEP after sexual intercourse. No convincing randomized controlled trials have been published (the best sort of evidence of efficacy).

Current guidelines are based on scientific plausibility and best-practice evidence and, in the UK, the drug regimens are based on those recommended by the Chief Medical Officer in the Department of Health's guidelines on occupational exposure, 2000.

Indirect evidence suggesting that PEP may be effective comes from three sources:

1. A retrospective case-control study in which health-care workers with needlestick exposure to HIV who were given zidovudine had an 81 per cent reduction in seroconversion compared with those who were not treated.

2. Animal studies using macaque monkeys.

3. Mother to child transmission of HIV in pregnancy suggests that much of the benefit of antiretroviral therapy is due to a PEP effect provided to the baby.

PEP should therefore be thought of as an unproven clinical intervention and its use should be considered on a case-by-case basis when:

the source is known or suspected to be HIV-positive;

significant exposure has occurred by direct contact of the vagina, anus, mouth or eye with semen, vaginal secretions or blood with or without tissue damage;

therapy can be initiated quickly and adherence to the regimen is likely.

## Should treatment be given in confirmed primary HIV infection?

There are arguments for and against use of drug treatment at this very early stage in HIV infection. It has been hypothesized that treating at this stage could alter the natural history of the infection for the better, by preserving the body's immune response to HIV. However no studies, so far, have shown that there is any long-term clinical benefit in treating individuals at this stage when compared with deferring treatment until later. Another argument in favour is that during this period the individual has a high viral load and so is more infectious. Reducing this with drugs could reduce HIV onward transmission.

On the other hand, we have to take into account the potential side-effects of the drugs and the very real risk of the development of resistant virus if adherence to the medication is poor. Further, no guidelines exist as to the optimal duration of treatment. At present the jury remains out but seems to favour treatment in this setting only as part of a clinical trial to determine its efficacy. Someone illustrated the question neatly with an analogy of chocolate bars, of which there are only a limited number. Do you eat them now when your belly is full (your immune system is functioning well), or do you wait until you're hungry?

## How likely am I to catch HIV from someone who is positive?

Many different factors influence the likelihood of HIV transmission but it is possible to rank various activities in terms of risk, all else being equal. The rates will be affected by presence of STIs, ulcers and trauma associated, say, with assault. The infecting person's stage of disease will also influence risk. As seen above, if he or she is seroconverting, this risk will be much greater.

| | |
|---|---|
| Receptive anal intercourse | 1 in 30 to 1 in 125 |
| Needle sharing | 1 in 150 |
| Needlestick injury in health workers | 1 in 300 |
| Receptive vaginal intercourse | 1 in 500 to 1 in 2000 |
| Insertive anal or vaginal intercourse | 1 in 1000 to 1 in 5000 |
| Mucous membrane splash | 1 in 1000 |
| Oral sex: no data but likely to be | 1 in 1000 or lower |

## Testing for HIV

To test or not to test? Debate has rallied back and forth regarding this question ever since the blood test became available towards the end of

1984. Entrenchment occurred early on and the general view was *not* to test. There were genuine worries among people, in those days predominantly in the gay community, that they would be marginalized, victimized and treated badly at work.

Insurance companies upped the premiums for young single men and even to have taken a test, whatever the result, made you part of a high-risk group and therefore uninsurable. In the UK, with the government's general encouragement for everybody to test, the Association of British Insurers announced in 1989 that there would be no insurance premium penalties for those who tested. This remains true today.

One strong argument against testing was that there was little to be done if the test came back positive, so why bother? Today there is so much that can be done that anybody, literally, who has the slightest chance of being infected should test. Put simply, there are two sorts of HIV-positive persons in the West today: those who haven't tested and will die of AIDS and those who have tested and will die of old age.

The 'window-period' is the time between catching HIV and the blood test, which measures antibodies, becoming positive. For years this has been taken as being up to three months. After this interval infection is deemed not to have happened and in many cases people have been advised to wait the full three months before testing. Today's HIV tests look, in addition to antibody, for the presence of antigen, bits of the virus itself, which is likely to be found earlier than the antibody. We believe that early diagnosis is a good thing, if only because extra precautions can be taken sooner not to pass on the virus, and we advise the taking of an HIV test earlier, even as little as two weeks after risk, as well as at three months.

## Case history

John P was a 55-year-old office worker who turned up at his local accident and emergency department complaining of tiredness, weight loss and shortness of breath. His wife and two grown-up children had come with him. He had a high temperature and a dry cough. On further questioning it seemed that he hadn't felt very well for many months. He had gradually begun to feel more tired and had noticed his trousers were getting loose. He was clearly unwell and, when admitted, was found to have low levels of oxygen in his blood as well as a high fever. Pneumonia was diagnosed and antibiotics were started. These seemed to have little effect and his condition deteriorated. When the chest X-ray was reviewed, one of his doctors said it looked like a fungal infection and was there any chance of an underlying immune suppression such as HIV?

> The doctors raised this possibility with John who then mentioned that he and his wife had not had sex for many years but that he had occasionally had sex with men. After pre-test counselling, an HIV test was performed which was positive. With appropriate treatment he made a very good recovery from his pneumocystis pneumonia (PCP) and was discharged ten days later with outpatient follow-up. He started antiretroviral therapy three weeks later. He told his wife of his diagnosis and she underwent testing and was found to be negative.

## Monitoring/tests including CD4 and viral load

Before we start, some of the terms need explaining: The *CD4 count* refers to the number of CD4 T-helper lymphocytes, one of the cells originally infected by HIV (see previous chapter). It is expressed as number of cells per cubic millimetre, say 700/mm$^3$. In general, the higher, the better. The *viral load* is a fairly accurate way of measuring the actual number of virus particles in the blood (or other fluid). It is a measure of HIV RNA and is expressed in copies per millilitre, say 50/ml or more often, a 'viral load of 50'. A viral load of 50 is better than a viral load of 50 000.

The aim of HIV management is to keep the patient well. After the diagnosis of HIV has been made (including a mandatory repeat confirmatory HIV antibody test) patients are seen in the outpatient clinic every 3–6 months. At these visits the patient's emotional and physical welfare are assessed and routine blood tests are taken. These include the CD4 count and the viral load, both of which measure the state of the immune system. These are called surrogate markers and are very important as patients can have advanced immune damage and no symptoms. The CD4 count tells us the current state of the immune system, whereas the viral load can be visualized more as a 'speedometer', that is, the higher the viral load the faster a person might progress on their journey with HIV.

In a healthy person without HIV infection, the CD4 count ('T'-cell count) is 500–1400 and the viral load is zero (they are not infected). A CD4 count of less than 200 represents severe immunosuppression and renders the patient susceptible to serious opportunistic infections, so-called because they do not cause illness in an individual with a fully functioning immune system.

## The natural history of HIV infection

Treatments have progressed so much over the past ten years that HIV, in many cases, has become more like a chronic medical problem akin to such conditions as diabetes mellitus.

The rate of progression of HIV varies between individuals for a number of reasons, many of which are unclear but include the severity of the primary infection, lifestyle factors and the type of HIV virus acquired. However, the average time from infection to profound immunosuppression is ten years. The stages of infection are listed below.

## Asymptomatic HIV infection

This is the period when a person has HIV but has no symptoms or outward signs that show that they are infected and they feel well. This can last for many months to years. The CD4 count during this time may well be above 350 but, as stated above, the immune system can become dangerously low during this time, without the patient developing symptoms, so it is imperative that the patient attends their 3–6-monthly review. This allows the progress of HIV to be monitored in the individual and treatment offered as soon as it is indicated.

As well as regular monitoring, general measures to optimize health and wellbeing are important which include stopping smoking. Long term use of certain herbal remedies, including echinacea, astragalus and ginseng, should be avoided in people living with HIV. While these substances are all 'immune enhancers', they can stimulate the wrong parts of the immune system in HIV-positive people and can actually enhance virus replication.

Co-infection with hepatitis B or C and HIV alters progression of each virus. Testing for these infections is imperative and vaccination for hepatitis A and B should be undertaken (if there is no evidence of previous infection).

Risk reduction methods should be advised not only to avoid hepatitis C but other STIs, other strains of HIV virus and forward transmission of the persons HIV virus.

As we have said, the aim of managing anyone with HIV is to prevent them becoming unwell. Although not everyone agrees, the general consensus, on a risk/benefit analysis, suggests that treatment is not warranted in an asymptomatic patient with a CD4 count of more than 350.

### Case history

Susan H was a 30-year-old woman who presented to the antenatal clinic when she was 14 weeks pregnant. She had been diagnosed HIV-positive 5 years previously when she tested following her ex-boyfriend's death from an AIDS defining condition. It was more than 10 years since she had shared needles with him – the distant past now – and she had not injected drugs since. Her CD4 count had always been good with her latest being over 500 and a viral load of 2000 (low).

She told the antenatal team about her diagnosis. Care was co-ordinated between the midwife, her obstetrician and her HIV doctor. As her immune system was functioning well, it was decided that she didn't need anti-HIV drugs for her own health but, in the second half of her pregnancy, antiretroviral therapy (ARV) was started to reduce the risk of transmission to her baby. She commenced taking treatment at week 24, a date was planned for her caesarean section and it was explained she shouldn't breast feed. The baby was to be given ARV for the first 6 weeks of its life.

The pregnancy went well as did the caesarean section at 38 weeks. Now at 3 months on the baby has had the 'all clear' and is definitely not infected. Susan H remains well; she stopped her medication after the birth and, as yet, has not needed treatment for her own infection.

## Symptomatic HIV infection

The first signs of HIV are often minor and varied. As a result, patients can present to GPs or other specialists with a wide variety of symptoms and it is not immediately apparent that HIV is the underlying diagnosis. The CD4 count is often 200–350 during this time. Common conditions include oral candida (thrush), persistent skin complaints including eczema, seborrhoeic dermatitis, warts and herpes, recurrent chest infections and mouth ulcers, night sweats, weight loss, gum disease and fatigue.

Good treatment is available for each of these specific conditions and we recommend regular dentist/hygienist appointments for the gum and tooth complaints. In addition, however, the time has now come to address the underlying immunosuppression and antiretroviral treatment should be commenced, depending on the CD4 count and the severity of symptoms.

As the symptoms relating to HIV can be so non-specific, it is important to investigate further for other possible underlying causes. Common conditions such as recurrent herpes can be treated with daily aciclovir, dry skin with antifungal creams and oral thrush with antifungal tablets or suspension. In a patient with a CD4 count of 350–200, treatment for HIV is discussed and should be started before the CD4 falls below 200. The different sorts of antiretroviral treatment are discussed below.

## Late HIV infection

Under this heading comes advanced HIV disease when immunosuppression had become marked. If a patient's CD4 count is less than 200 this renders them at high risk of an opportunistic infection (OI) or tumour. The term 'AIDS' is used when one of these conditions is present. In the old days before HAART, an AIDS diagnosis indicated a very poor prognosis and, if not imminent death, at least severe ill-health.

There are many opportunistic infections, the commonest being PCP (*Pneumocystis carinii* pneumonia). This is a fungal infection affecting the lungs. It presents with a dry cough, fevers, weight loss and shortness of breath on exertion. The symptoms can vary in severity but are often insidious in onset and gradually worsen if treatment isn't instigated. Incidentally, the 'C' in PCP has recently been renamed '*jiroveci*' but 'PJP' has yet to catch on and we prefer the old name.

There are also a number of opportunistic tumours including lymphoma and Kaposi's sarcoma (KS). KS was an AIDS defining diagnosis in 30 per cent of patients in the 1980s but the incidence has since fallen. It is associated with human herpes virus 8 (HHV-8). It can affect any part of the body but commonly presents with distinctive dusky red papules on the skin. Treatment for the underlying HIV may be enough but local radiotherapy or chemotherapy is sometimes needed.

## Management of late HIV infection

Any patient presenting with a possible AIDS-defining condition needs urgent investigation and management and this often warrants hospital admission. The underlying condition, PCP for example, needs confirming with tests and then fully treating *before* any anti-HIV treatment is commenced. This is because improving the immune system with HAART in these immediate circumstances can do more harm than good. The opportunistic infection can, paradoxically, actually be worsened by restoring the immune system. Once the OI has been treated *then* HAART is started (an interval of about three weeks depending on individual circumstances).

## The multidisciplinary approach

In the post-HAART era, the management of HIV has markedly altered. Indeed, since 1997 the outlook and prognosis of those with HIV has become much more favourable and the mortality rate has fallen. Centres looking after HIV-infected individuals have made many adaptations to their services as a result.

It is important to remember to see the person as a whole and address all aspects of their physical and emotional wellbeing which includes their sex life. This doesn't just mean screening for STIs and advising no unprotected sex. It means helping people to adjust to their diagnosis and enabling them to deal with issues that it frequently poses.

The model of care, in HIV centres, is very much multidisciplinary. The team is comprised of many individuals including specialist HIV pharmacists, adherence nurses, research nurses, dieticians, midwives, counsellors and strong links with the GUM clinic, support groups and local advice centres for help with such issues as housing and immigration.

In many centres, the San Francisco General Hospital's approach of on-site availability of other specialties hugely improves the quality of care. Eye, chest and skin specialists, neurologists, ENT surgeons and dentists all have their part to play.

# Treatment – antiretroviral therapy

## NRTIs

The oldest class of drugs are the nucleoside reverse transcriptase inhibitors (NRTIs) which include zidovudine, didanosine and lamivudine.

The first drug used for the treatment of HIV was zidovudine (AZT) in the mid 1980s. This was a drug that had lain unused on a pharmaceutical company's shelves for many years having originally been developed as an anti-cancer therapy. Although it was slightly worrying that the reason zidovudine had never been made available was on account of its bad side-effects, it was, nonetheless, shown at the time to be better than placebo in symptomatic individuals. For many years this was the only specific anti-HIV drug available. Although it was not possible to measure at the time, this use of a solitary antiretroviral was a recipe for resistance to develop in HIV and this undoubtedly occurred, probably within a year of treatment starting. However, for all its drawbacks, AZT provided the first glimmer of hope and certainly prolonged life, albeit for a short time.

Zidovudine worked by stopping the activity of HIV's special intracellular enzyme, reverse transcriptase (see previous chapter). The search was on for other NRTIs and, once found, monotherapy, the use of one antiretroviral, was replaced by dual therapy (zidovudine with didanosine, lamivudine or zalcitibine). These combinations, in a three-year follow-up period, were shown to reduce mortality by 36 per cent.

A more recent addition to this class is emtricitabine (FTC). Tenofovir is a nucleotide reverse transcriptase inhibitor which works in a similar way to NNRTIs (see below).

## NNRTIs

Non-nucleoside reverse transcriptase inhibitors (NNRTIs) comprise a class of drugs that only work on HIV-1, not HIV-2. There are two drugs in this class: efavirenz and nevirapine. Both can be given once daily and trials have shown no difference in efficacy. Resistance to this class of drugs is mediated by a single virus mutation which means that if you fail on one of these drugs the virus will also be resistant to the other drug.

With the arrival of this second class of drugs, the era of triple therapy had begun. The use of two NRTIs and one NNRTI made tight control of HIV infection possible, but not for everyone. HIV is capable of changing and developing resistance very rapidly. Nevirapine, for example, becomes rapidly useless on its own or as one of a pair. It was not very effective when used on those who had already developed resistance to other antiretrovirals. This is one of the most important messages of HIV therapy. *Every effort must be made to prevent resistance developing*. This means that adequate levels of drug must be given and treatment must be taken without fail.

Easy enough, you might think, but in the early days of triple therapy there was a real burden simply in managing to take all the drugs (more than thirty a day in some cases) on some regimens. In others, the side-effects were really hard to put up with.

## Protease inhibitors

In 1996, yet another class of drugs was introduced, the protease inhibitors, which bind to one of the virus's enzymes and stop further viruses being produced. They were initially difficult to take, with a high pill burden, numerous side-effects and dietary restrictions but despite this they had a massive effect on survival. There are many drugs in this class and, over time, they have improved with regard to ease of administration and reduction in side-effects. Examples include lopinavir and ritonavir. The newest of the protease inhibitors is atazanavir which is licensed for once-daily use.

With this now quite large selection of antiretrovirals available, it has become possible to tailor treatment to specific clinical scenarios.

Apart from these three major classes of drugs, there exist two other types of agent. The first is a fusion inhibitor (enfurvitide), a twice-daily injection that works by preventing HIV from entering cells. Another group of new drugs, currently undergoing clinical trials with encouraging results, are the CCR5 inhibitors.

## Principles of treatment

HIV replicates at a rate of approximately $10^9$ viral particles a day. This rapid turnover leads to mutations in the virus which provides the mechanism for production of resistance to certain drugs. In 1997 the concept of 'highly active antiretroviral therapy' was born. This used the principle of combining three different drugs from two different classes which made it more difficult for the highly suppressed virus to make enough mutations to evade the effect of the drugs. Most drug combinations now are once or twice-daily regimes.

The most important aspect of treatment is adherence. If the level of the drugs in the blood is low this can lead to failure of inhibition of viral replication. This in turn can lead to resistance to the drugs and failure of that specific regime. Studies have shown that adherence needs to be better than 95 per cent. This means that over 95 per cent of the time the person has to take the right dose at the right time. CD4 counts and viral loads are measured a number of times over the first three months. The viral load should then have reduced to less than 50 copies/ml. Subsequent bloods are taken every three months thereafter. These are not only to monitor the CD4 and viral load but kidney, liver, lipid and glucose tests to check for adverse effects of the drugs.

## Side-effects

Different classes of drugs have their own specific side-effects as do different drugs in each class. General effects of NRTIs include nausea, vomiting, abdominal pain, changes in body shape due to fat being laid down in the wrong places (lipodystrophy) and headaches. Protease inhibitors are often associated with diarrhoea, lipodystrophy, glucose and lipid abnormalities. NNRTIs commonly cause a rash; efavirenz can cause vivid dreams, insomnia and depression; nevirapine can cause liver abnormalities and a serious hypersensitivity (allergic) reaction.

It is important when starting any new drug to be aware that it can cause side-effects and to seek medical opinion if you suspect this. The aim of HIV treatment is to give someone a good and long quality of life. Patients should no longer be expected to suffer unmanageable side-effects. If these don't settle down or are intolerable (or are serious), then the drugs can be changed. We expect to be able to find a combination for each person, which, after the first few weeks, will have no or minimal side-effects.

# Resistance testing

This is an important investigation performed on an individual's personal virus to see whether it is resistant to any drugs. 'Primary resistance' is the term used when a person is initially infected with HIV that is resistant to certain drugs, even though that person has never had any antiretroviral treatment. It means that the person from whom the infection was acquired already had, themselves, a resistant strain of HIV. This occurs in approximately 10–15 per cent of transmissions.

Every new patient diagnosed with HIV has resistance testing done to guide the choice of drug to be used if or when they need treatment. The other setting in which this test is crucial is when a person is taking antiretrovirals but the treatment appears to be failing, for example when the viral load is no longer undetectable despite taking the drugs. This helps the next combination to be planned accurately.

# Clinical trials

As with all specialties of medicine, clinical trials are performed in the field of HIV. Most large HIV centres have their own research unit incorporated into their clinical department which employ doctors and research nurses. As you will have read we now have drugs that provide effective treatment for the treatment of HIV. For this reason, potential new drugs are not compared with placebo but with the current gold standard, the best treatment available. New drugs will have gone through extensive trials before they ever appear at the phase that involves patients.

Trials these days are used not only to look at new drugs but also to answer important and topical questions such as 'How beneficial is treatment in primary HIV infection?'; 'Can patients safely have a break from their treatment?'; 'What is the rate of heart disease in HIV-positive patients and what effect do HIV drugs have on this?' Also under investigation are potential HIV vaccines both preventative, to stop the virus being caught in the first place, and therapeutic, to slow down progression of the diseases in those already infected.

Strategies for Management of Antiretroviral Therapy (SMART) is one example of a new long-term study and is currently being organized by, among others, the National Institutes of Health (NIH) in the USA and the Medical Research Council (MRC) in the UK. This will involve about 6000 people enrolled over three or so years who will then be either offered immediate antiviral therapy, the *Go* group, or will be carefully monitored until (as is normal practice these days) the CD4 count falls when they will be given treatment, the *Wait* group. Both groups will be followed for between six and nine years.

Why would anyone want to take part in studies such as this? Well, there are the general benefits to other HIV-positive people, in this case by suggesting which of these perfectly reasonable strategies is preferable, or whether there is no difference. Secondly, those who take part in the study will benefit from extra close attention over the period of the trial.

Any proposed trial is rigorously examined regarding its ethical status and all projects have to gain local ethics board approval. In the setting of trials in developing countries there is no exception and drug companies have to adhere to strict guidelines which include, for example, an undertaking to provide their drugs for the study patients, lifelong, not just for the duration of the trial.

## Resources

Terence Higgins Trust

www.aidsmap.com

www.i-base.info

www.bhiva.org

www.bodyandsoul.demon.co.uk

www.positivelywomen.org.uk

www.womenhiv.org

www.nat.org.uk

# glossary of terms

**Abscess**  A walled-in collection of pus.

**Acute**  Early (in the course of a disease), relatively severe, sharp; opposite of chronic.

**AIN**  Anal Intraepithelial Neoplasia.

**Aneurysm**  a dilatation in the wall of an artery.

**Anterior**  In front of.

**Antibiotic**  A chemical substance capable of killing or preventing the growth of bacteria.

**Antibody**  A protein elaborated by the body's defence mechanisms which neutralizes specific 'foreign' substances (antigens), such as bacteria or viruses.

**Antifungal**  A chemical substance capable of killing or preventing the growth of yeasts or fungi.

**Antigen**  Any substance which, when introduced into the body, stimulates the production of antibodies.

**Antiviral**  A chemical substance capable of killing or preventing the growth of viruses.

**Anvil syndrome**  Deep dyspareunia as a result of ovary being banged against the pelvic wall.

**Arthritis**  Inflammation of one or more joints. May occur in chlamydial infection, gonorrhoea and syphilis.

**Axilla**  The armpit.

**Bacterium**  Bacteria are tiny, one-celled organisms that include the causes of gonorrhoea, chlamydial infection, LGV, chancroid, Donovanosis, and syphilis. They are usually amenable to treatment with antibiotics.

**Balanitis**  Inflammation of the foreskin.

**Balano-posthitis** inflammation of the foreskin and glans penis.

**Bartholin's glands** Two glands situated at the lower third of the labia which secrete a thin mucus to aid lubrication during sexual intercourse. The ducts may become blocked leading to painful swelling – Bartholinitis.

**Bejel** One of the tropical treponematoses.

**Biopsy** Surgical removal of a piece of tissue for laboratory examination.

**Bubo** Swelling of a lymph node due to infection, particularly in the axilla or groin, as in LGV or chancroid.

*Candida Albicans* A yeast-like fungus responsible for thrush, vaginal discharge and balano-posthitis.

**Cardiovascular** Referring to the heart and blood vessels.

**Carrier** Someone infected by a microorganism who shows no sign of the infection, but is infectious to others.

**Cerebro-spinal fluid** The liquid that bathes the brain and spinal cord.

**Cervix** From the Latin for neck, it refers to the vaginal portion of the uterus. Infection or inflammation of the cervix is called cervicitis.

**Chancre** The sore, usually painless, found in early syphilis.

**Chancroid** The tropical STI causing painful sores on the genitalia.

**Chronic** Long-standing; the opposite of acute.

**CIN** Cervical intraepithelial neoplasia. Term for pre-cancerous changes on a cervical biopsy. Being replaced by SIL.

**Clitoris** The sensitive, erectile organ in women, equivalent to the glans penis.

**Coccus** A round bacterium. In gonorrhoea the organisms come in pairs, *diplo*-cocci.

**Commensal** A microorganism that lives in or on the body without causing disease. *Candida Albicans* is found in a majority of people's intestines as a Commensal.

**Condylomata acuminata** Genital warts, caused by HPV. Not to be confused with:

**Condylomata lata** The highly infectious wart-like growths found around the anus (and other moist body areas) in secondary syphilis.

**Congenital** Present at birth having been acquired during pregnancy.

**Conjunctivitis** Inflammation or infection of the covering of the eye and lining of the eyelid.

**Crabs** Infestation with pubic lice.

**Culture** The process of growing microorganisms in the laboratory to aid their identification.

**Cunnilingus** Oral stimulation of the female genitalia.

**Cutaneous** Referring to the skin.

**Cyst** A sac, often containing fluid.

**Cystitis** Infection or inflammation of the bladder.

**Dermatitis** Inflammation of the skin.

**Disseminated Gonococcal Infection** (DGI) Spread of gonococcal infection to other parts (usually joints and skin).

**Discharge** an excretion of fluid or pus, usually from the vagina or urethra.

**Donavanosis** A tropical or sub-tropical sexually transmitted disease.

**Dysentery** Bacterial infection of the intestine, occasionally followed by SARA.

**Dysmenorrhoea** Pain at the time of the menstrual period.

**Dyspareunia** Pain felt by the woman during sexual intercourse. It may be superficial when there is infection of the vulva, or deep, as in salpingitis.

**Dysuria** Pain or discomfort on passing urine.

**Ectopic** In the wrong place. Used to describe a pregnancy when the fertilized egg has implanted outside the uterus, often in the fallopian tubes.

**Elephantiasis** Swelling of tissue following blockage of lymphatics; occurs in LGV.

**Endocarditis** Infection of the heart valves, seen very rarely with gonorrhoea.

**Endometrium** The blood-rich lining of the uterus which, if pregnancy does not occur, is shed each month as the menstrual flow.

**Endemic** A steady and constant state of infection in a community varying little year by year.

**Enzyme** A biologically active protein that helps chemical reactions (like digestion).

**Epidemic** An increasing level of infection in a community.

**Epidemiological treatment** The giving of antibiotics before, or without, confirmation of a diagnosis.

**Epidemiology** The study of patterns of disease.

**Epididymis** the coiled first part of the tube connecting the testis, via the seminal vesicles, to the urethra.

**Epithelium**  The layer of cells covering other tissue. Skin and mucous membrane are examples.

**Erosion**  Literally an 'eating-away' or ulcer of an epithelium. When the usual epithelium of the outside of the cervix is replaced by that from inside the cervix, the appearance is sometimes described as an erosion. Quite normal.

**Exudate**  A fluid 'oozed' out, like sweat. Due to inflammation it may contain many white blood cells. The urethral discharge in gonorrhoea is an exudate.

**Fallopian Tube**  These connect the ovaries and the uterus. Infection in the tubes is called salpingitis.

**Fellatio**  Oral stimulation of the penis.

**Fitzhugh-Curtis syndrome**  Perihepatitis, where gonorrhoea or chlamydial infection has spread to involve the lining of the liver.

**Fistula**  A canal or track connecting an internal organ with another or with the outside world. Usually the result of disease.

**Foreskin**  the retractable skin which covers the glans penis. Removed at circumcision.

**Frei test**  A skin test used in the diagnosis of LGV. Rarely performed today.

**Frequency (of micturition)**  Passing urine more often than usual. It may be during the day (diurnal), nocturnal, or both. It is more often a symptom of cystitis than of sexually transmitted disease.

**FTA-Abs test**  short for the fluorescent treponemal antibody absorbed test, a specific blood-test for treponemal disease.

**Fungi**  These are vegetable organisms of a low order of development. Although mushrooms, toadstools, and moulds are more familiar, there are several fungi pathogenic to man. *Candida albicans* is the most ubiquitous of these.

**Genito-urinary**  Referring to the reproductive and excretory systems. The latter with reference to the kidneys, bladder, etc.

**Genitourinary Medicine**  The new name for the specialty of Venereology encompassing a broader vision of sexual health.

**Gland**  An organ that secretes a substance. The term is loosely used to describe the lymph nodes which are found throughout the body. 'Swollen glands' implies infection.

**Gonococcus**  *Neisseria gonorrhoeae,* the bacterium responsible for gonorrhoea. It is a gram-negative coccus.

**Gonorrhoea** The commonest of the 'true' venereal diseases. Characterized by dysuria and urethral discharge in men and few symptoms in women.

**Gram-stain** A method of staining micro-organisms to facilitate their microscopic examination and identification.

**Gumma** The inflammatory tumour or infiltration found in tertiary syphilis.

**HAART** Highly Active AntiRetroviral Therapy, a combination treatment for HIV infection utilising at least three different drugs.

**Herpes simplex** The virus responsible for 'cold sores'. Type I is usually responsible for infection of the mouth and lips, while type II more often affects the genitalia.

**HPV** Human Papilloma Virus, the cause of warts.

**Hutchinson's triad** Three stigmata of congenital syphilis: Hutchinson's teeth, nerve deafness, and interstitial keratitis, a clouding of the front of the eye.

**Hypertrophy** An increase in the size of an organ or tissue.

**Incidence** The number of cases occurring in a defined area during a specified period of time.

**Incubation period** The time between acquiring an infection and developing signs or symptoms.

**Indurated** Hard.

**Infectivity** The likelihood of a given infection being passed on to those exposed to it. Very few infections have an infectivity of 100 per cent. The infectivity of most sexually transmitted diseases is unknown.

**Inflammation** The reaction of tissues to injury or infection. Inflammation is characterized by pain, swelling, redness, and warmth. White cells are attracted to areas of inflammation.

**Inguinal** Referring to the groin region.

**Intracellular** Literally 'inside a cell'. A requirement for the diagnosis of gonorrhoea using the microscope.

**Introitus** The entrance to the vagina.

*In vitro* Referring to the results of tests or experiments in the laboratory in test-tubes or other apparatus, in contrast to

*In vivo* which refers to the effects of such tests in living animals or humans.

**Iritis** Inflammation of the iris or the eye.

**Jarisch-Herxheimer reaction**  A reaction that follows the start of treatment for syphilis perhaps caused by the break-up of the bacteria responsible. There is a brief flu-like illness and syphilitic lesions may get temporarily worse.

**Koilocytosis**  Wart infection of the cervix which shows up on cervical cytology, the 'smear test'.

**Labia**  The lips around the vagina. Labia minora are the small lips surrounding the introitus, and outside these are the larger labia majora.

**Labial**  Confusingly, usually refers to the lips around the mouth. Thus labial herpes is an infection on the face rather than the genitalia.

**Latent**  Hidden or concealed. Often refers to the presence of a disease which doesn't show itself.

**Lateral**  At the side, or to the side of.

**Lesion**  A local wound or disruption of tissue. The result of a pathological process or trauma.

**Leucocyte**  A white blood-cell.

**Lues**  An old-fashioned word for syphilis.

**Lymphadenopathy**  A swelling of the lymph nodes.

**Lymphocyte**  A sort of white cell formed in the lymph glands, concerned with immunity and antibody production.

**Lymphogranuloma venereum** (LGV)  A tropical or sub-tropical sexually transmitted disease caused by *Chlamydia trachomatis.*

**Lumbar puncture**  A procedure in which the cerebro-spinal fluid is sampled to ascertain whether infection is involving the central nervous system.

**Macule**  A discoloured spot on the skin, not raised above the normal surface. A macule may evolve into a papule, vesicle, or pustule.

**Macrolyde**  A group of antibiotics including erythromycin and azithromycin. Effective against many STIs.

**Medium**  The substance on which micro-organisms may be cultured in the laboratory.

**Meningitis**  Inflammation (usually infection) of the meninges, which are the layers surrounding the brain and spinal cord. Meningitis occurs in secondary syphilis and rarely in gonorrhoea.

**Menstruation**  The monthly loss of Endometrium from the uterus. The 'period'.

**Metronidazole**  A drug useful against *Trichomonas vaginalis* and certain anaerobic bacteria (those that do not like oxygen).

**Micturition**  Passing urine.

**Mucous membrane**  The shiny epithelium lining the cavities of the body open to the air, such as the mouth, respiratory tract, and genitalia.

**Neonatal**  Referring to the period soon after birth.

**Neoplasm**  A tumour or new growth.

**Neurosyphilis**  The involvement of the nervous system by syphilis. The best known manifestations are tabes dorsalis and general paralysis of the insane (GPI).

**Nodule**  Small palpable swelling, usually in the skin.

**Non-specific urethritis (NSU)**  Also known as non-gonococcal urethritis (NGU), this is the most common form of urethritis.

**Oedema**  Swelling due to retention of fluid.

**Ophthalmia neonatorum**  Infection of the eye of the newborn baby. The gonococcus used to be the most common cause, more recently chlamydia has been implicated in many cases.

**Orchitis**  Inflammation or infection of the testis.

**Ovary**  The paired female sex gland which produces the ovum and also makes sex hormones.

**Palpable**  Discernible by touch.

**Pandemic**  A disease that has spread all over the world.

**Papule**  A skin lesion raised above the surface.

**Parasite**  A plant or animal that lives on or within another organism at the expense of that organism.

**Pathogen**  A micro-organism capable of producing disease.

**Pelvic inflammatory disease (PID)**  Infection of the pelvic organs in the female, often used synonymously with salpingitis.

**Penicillin**  The first antibiotic. Still the first line of treatment for syphilis.

**Peri-anal**  Around the anus.

**Perineum**  The area of skin between the anus and the vagina, in women, and the scrotum, in men.

**Peritonitis**  Infection involving the lining of the abdominal organs, the peritoneum. Often associated with acute appendicitis, it may complicate salpingitis if this is not treated early.

**pH**  A measure of the acidity of a fluid. pH 7 is neutral; the lower the pH, the more acid.

**Pharynx**  The throat.

**Phimosis**  A constriction of the foreskin preventing it from being drawn back over the Penis. Occasionally, having been retracted, the foreskin cannot be brought forward again. This is called paraphimosis. Both these conditions are sometimes brought on as a result of sexually transmitted disease.

**PIN**  Penile Intraepithelial Neoplasia, changes similar to CIN occurring on the penis.

**Pinta**  A tropical treponemal disease caused by *Treponema careatum*. Not sexually transmitted.

**Placebo**  The inactive substance given when assessing the efficacy of a treatment.

**Placenta**  The organ separating the maternal from the foetal circulation in the uterus, while allowing the transfer of nutrients and oxygen and the elimination of waste material; the afterbirth.

**Polymorphonuclear leucocyte**  The white blood-cell that is responsible for the formation of pus, hence its common name, the 'pus' cell. It is phagocytic, that is it can ingest bacteria and other debris.

**Posterior**  Behind, at the back of.

**Prevalence**  The number of cases of a disease in an area at a given point in time.

**Proctitis**  Inflammation or infection of the rectum. Common among male homosexuals, it may be caused by the gonococcus or may be a manifestation of non-gonococcal infection.

**Prostatitis**  Inflammation or infection of the prostate gland.

**Protozoon**  A large single-celled organism. *Trichomonas vaginalis* is a protozoon.

**Pruritus**  Itchiness or irritation.

**Purulent**  Made up of pus.

**Pustule**  A raised spot on the skin containing pus.

**Reagin**  A group of antibodies which increase in quantity when there is active syphilis. It is reagin that is measured by the non-specific blood-tests such as the WR or the VDRL.

**Reiter's disease**  See SARA.

**Rhagades**  Small linear scars around the corners of the mouth seen in some patients with congenital syphilis.

**Rod**  A long bacterium. The causative organism of chancroid is a rod.

**Salpingitis**  Infection of the fallopian tubes. Gonorrhoea used to be the most common cause but is now isolated in well under 50 per cent of cases.

**SARA** Sexually Acquired Reactive Arthritis is the modern term for those cases of Reiter's disease or syndrome following infection with *Chlamydia trachomatis*. Typically there is a urethritis, arthritis, conjunctivitis, and skin lesions.

**Scabies (the itch)** A contagious skin disease caused by a mite, *Sarcoptes scabiei*.

**Seminal vesicle** A small secretory sac attached to the vas deferens.

**Septicaemia** The presence of bacterial toxins in the blood.

**Serological tests for syphilis (STS)** The blood tests used to diagnose syphilis. They include the reagin tests as well as the specific tests.

**Serum** The portion of blood left after the solid components have been removed. Also describes the exudate from a chancre, which can be examined microscopically.

**SIL** Squamous Intraepithelial Lesion, a replacement for CIN.

**Sinus** A hollow space or channel usually caused by a pathological process.

**Slide** The glass microscope slide on which material from potentially infected sites is placed prior to staining and examination.

**Snuffles** The heavy watery discharge from the nose and pharynx of the new-born child with congenital syphilis. The exudate is teeming with treponemes.

**Spirochaete** A member of the genus to which *Treponema pallidum* belongs.

**Stat** To be given at once (of medicines).

**Stricture** An abnormal narrowing in a tube or channel. Urethral stricture is one of the late complications of untreated gonorrhoea in the male.

**Suppuration** The formation of pus, usually leading to its discharge as from an abscess.

**Syphilis** One of the oldest of the venereal diseases, caused by *Treponema pallidum*.

**Systemic** Not localized, involving the whole of the body.

**Testis** The paired male sex gland, which produces spermatazoa and the male sex hormones.

**Tetracycline** Like penicillin, an antibiotic, but one that is active against a wider variety of bacteria. A useful treatment for NSU.

**Thrombosis** The development of a clot or thrombus in a blood vessel.

**Titre**  The measure of the amount of antibody present in the blood by a method of dilution.

**TPHA, TPPA and TPI**  Specific blood tests for the detection of syphilis.

**Trauma**  A wound or injury, not necessarily of a severe nature.

*Treponema pallidum*  The causative organism of syphilis.

*Trichomonas vaginalis*  The protozoon responsible for a vaginal infection in women and a low-grade urethritis in men.

**Urethra**  The tube connecting the bladder with the outside world.

**Urethritis**  inflammation or infection in the urethra.

**Urgency**  The feeling of need to pass water immediately.

**Uterus**  The womb. The organ in which the foetus develops.

**Vagina**  The channel through which childbirth takes place and entered by the erect penis during sexual intercourse.

**Vaginitis**  Inflammation of the vagina. Most often due to *Candida albicans,* although other organisms, particularly trichomonas, may be responsible.

**Vas deferens**  The tube connecting the testis to the urethra.

**Virus**  The smallest of the micro-organisms to affect man. They are not susceptible to antibiotics.

**Venereal**  Having to do with sex; from Venus, the goddess of love.

**VDRL**  The Venereal Disease Reference Laboratory blood test, one of the easiest and cheapest of the non-specific blood-tests for syphilis.

**Vesicle**  A small blister. Characteristic of herpetic infection at an early stage.

**VIN**  Vulval Intraepithelial Neoplasia, changes similar to CIN occurring on the vulva.

**Vulva**  The female external genital area.

**Vulvovaginitis**  Inflammation of the vulva and vagina together.

**Warts**  Transmissible skin growths caused by human papilloma virus.

**Wasserman Reaction (WR)**  The first blood-test used for the diagnosis of syphilis in the first decade of the last century. Now superseded by more modern tests.

**Yaws**  A treponemal disease of tropical climes caused by *Treponema pertenue.* It is not sexually transmitted.

# index

Note: Entries in the glossary section have not been indexed.

usefulness of a test, numbers
    affecting 19
worldwide situation 21
reverse transcriptase 130
rhagades 106
ribavirin 126
ribonucleic acid (RNA) 130
ritonavir 153


*Salmonella* 66
salmonellosis 121
salpingitis 69, 70
samples 5–6, 14
*Sarcoptes scabeii see* scabies
'saxophone penis' 112
scabies (*Sarcoptes scabeii*) 1, 115–16,
    118–20
sebaceous cysts 93–4
'senile' atrophy 37–8
sensitivity 17–19, 71
seroconversion 144
sexually acquired reactive arthritis
    (SARA) 66, 67
*Shigella* 66
shigellosis 121
side-effects 153, 154
'sign of the groove' 112, 114
simian immunodeficiency virus (SIV)
    129
skenitis 48
skin:
    conditions 36
    problems 66
    rash 103
    tags 94
smear test 4, 33, 96–7
specificity 17–19, 71
speculum examination 5, 6
spicy foods 51, 53
spots 117, 120–1
squamous intraepithelial lesions 96
*Staphylococcus aureus* 50
steroids 25, 28, 35, 36, 37, 108
'stigmata' 106
stress 83–4
sub-Saharan Africa 8, 13, 21, 111, 132,
    141

sulphonamides 49, 62
suppressive therapy 86
surgery 96
surveillance 14–15
syphilis 3, 4, 7, 9, 99–110, 137
    acquired 101, 102–5
    blood tests 3
    cardiovascular 104
    cases today 100–1
    causes 101
    congenital 101, 105–6
    diagnosis 101–2
    early stage 105, 108, 109, 144
    endemic 110
    historical aspects 99–100
    and HIV/AIDS 108–9
    late stage 105, 106, 108
    latent stage 104
    and lymphogranuloma venereum
        113
    national figures 21
    secondary stage 103, 109
    treatment 106
    treatment, evolution of 106–7
    treatment, modern 107–8
    tropical treponematoses 109–10
*see also* primary chancre


T-cells 131
tabes dorsalis 105
tampon 34
    retained 9
tenofovir 152
tests, reliability of 16
tetracyclines 61, 62, 74, 75, 108, 113,
    115
threadworms 10, 27, 122
throat 44, 45, 47
thrush 3, 4, 9, 10, 23, 25–8, 30,
    32, 37, 57
    complications 28
    and herpes simplex 83
    and non-specific genital infection
        59, 60
    and non-specific urethritis 56
    oral 150
    reasons for contracting 25–6